D1173511

essential ayurveda

essential ayurveda

what it is & what it can do for you

SHUBHRA KRISHAN

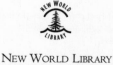

NEW WORLD LIBRARY
NOVATO, CALIFORNIA
www.newworldlibrary.com

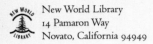New World Library
14 Pamaron Way
Novato, California 94949

Edited by Georgia A. Hughes and Katharine Farnam Conolly
Front cover design by Mary Beth Salmon
Text design and typography by Tona Pearce Myers

The material in this book is intended for education. It is not meant to take the place of diagnosis and treatment by a qualified medical practitioner or therapist. No expressed or implied guarantee as to the effects of the use of the recommendations can be given nor liability taken.

Grateful acknowledgment is given to Gopi Eberle and Mari Gayatri Stein for use of the yoga illustrations in chapter 12. Illustrations by Gopi Eberle from *Yoga Transformations* audiocassette by Mari Gayatri Stein. Copyright © 1984 by Mari Gayatri Stein. www.marigayatri.com

Library of Congress Cataloging-in-Publication Data
Krishan, Shubhra, 1966–
  Essential ayurveda : what it is & what it can do for you / by Shubhra Krishan.
      p.   cm.
Includes index.
  ISBN 1-57731-234-1 (pbk. : alk. paper)
  1. Medicine, Ayurvedic. I. Title.
  R605 .K725 2003
  615.5'3—dc21   2002014135

First Printing, February 2003
ISBN 1-57731-234-1
Printed in Canada on acid-free, partially recycled paper
Distributed to the trade by Publishers Group West

10 9 8 7 6 5 4 3 2

dedication

This work is dedicated to two of the most important people in my life: one who made me, and one who made it possible for me to realize my dream.

To my father, an ocean of insight. I stroll on the wind-washed shores of his memories, drinking in the knowledge and love he left me.

And, to Anandji, a mountain of inspiration, who will always tower on the horizon of my consciousness.

CONTENTS

acknowledgments

First and foremost, I have my mother to thank for raising me to believe in myself and always putting my needs before her own. How truly she lives up to her name "Mamta," which means "motherly love."

I am also deeply grateful to my brother, Sachin, for his you'd-better-write-a-book admonitions that finally worked; my husband, Hemant, for being my friend and unflattering critic; my son, Harshvardhan, and my dearest friends, Shirin, Chetna, Bena, Prita, and Sylvia, for filling my life with their affection; Vasu Nargundkar for her tips, advice, guidance, and tremendous support throughout the writing of this book; Vaidya Ramakant Mishra for sharing with me his infinite Ayurvedic wisdom; Bob Rose for his insights on yoga, and his generosity with resource material; Georgia Hughes for lifting my proposal off the slush pile, giving me this chance, and encouraging me throughout the writing of this book; and Katie Farnam Conolly for her incisive editing, kind words, and infinite patience.

the lunch that
changed my life

*It's a helluva start, being able to recognize
what makes you happy.*

— Lucille Ball, June 22, 1993

A Boeing 747 rises off the runway at London's Gatwick Airport. Gazing down at the rapidly diminishing carpet of cool green meadows, I feel my eyes mist over. It has been an exhilarating English summer, spent among beloved friends.

By contrast, walking through the hallway of New Delhi's Indira Gandhi International Airport is like swimming through a custard of melted sun. The heat threatens to liquefy my eyeballs inside their sockets. Every nerve in my skull is dissolving. But, ah, it is so good to be back home.

In the airport lounge, my mother wraps her soft arms around me, and I can smell mustard oil and curry leaves in her hair. Curry and rice — yum! My stomach rumbles happily in anticipation of the wonderful lunch awaiting me at my mother's home.

Each time I think back to that lunch, my heart fills with gratitude. Of course it was delicious, warm, welcoming. But what made it unforgettable was that it changed my life.

We had just sat down to lunch when the doorbell rang. An elderly man stood at the door, wearing a cotton kurta-pajama and an affable smile. My father introduced him as Vaidya Divakar Sharma, our new neighbor. Vaidya Sharma had stopped by to give my mother an herbal formulation for her cough, but at our insistence he stayed for lunch.

I was, of course, familiar with the word vaidya. It comes from the Sanskrit word *vid*, or "knowledge," and means "one who knows." I knew that Ayurvedic physicians were called vaidyas, but I had never met one before.

Over lunch, the vaidya remarked I looked more than exhausted from my journey; I looked unwell. "You look like you need some hydration therapy" were his exact words. "Really," I smiled politely, helping myself to another ladleful of curry.

By evening, I was decidedly ill: fever, shivering, abdominal cramps, and a horrible burning sensation in my urine. I rushed to the nearest hospital, and they diagnosed me with acute urinary tract infection.

The doctor advised me to stay off coffee and spices, and to start a seven-day course of Norfloxacin. And, yes, "Drink lots of water," he said.

Water. Hydration. The vaidya's words floated back into my consciousness. How had he known?

The next morning, I downed my first dose of antibiotic and phoned Vaidya Sharma for a formal appointment.

Sitting in his verandah-turned-clinic, the vaidya wore starched snow-white clothes reminiscent of the Ganges-bathing, mantra-chanting sadhus of the Himalayan foothills. His wife, pleasant and petite, brought me a tall glass of cool rose-water sherbet.

I opened my mouth to tell the vaidya about my condition, but his hand waved me into silence. Sitting close to me, he placed three delicate fingers on my wrist, supporting it with the ball of his thumb. Then he leaned back and closed his eyes. It was as if, in that one silent minute, he was drawing on his lifetime of training to hear the inside story of my body.

When Vaidya Divakar Sharma opened his eyes, he asked me an unexpected question: "Have you had persistent throat problems?" I nodded, stunned. He was right, but how could holding my wrist tell him about my throat? And weren't we supposed to be addressing a totally different region anyway?

As his fingers pressed slightly harder, his questions began to come more rapidly: "Do you tend to clench your teeth?" "Do you often miss lunch?" Then, most curiously — and accurately — "Do you have a tendency to suppress your real feelings most of the time?" I remember thinking what a Sherlock Holmes–like situation this was; here was a man I had barely met, piecing together fragments of my personality from clues I had no idea I was giving out.

Vaidya Sharma caught the questions as they darted from my eyes. Holmes would have chided Watson for his lack of perception. The vaidya only smiled. "It's really quite simple. The human pulse is intimately communicative, and we vaidyas are trained to pick up its signals, both superficial and deep. Ah, the things your pulse can tell me — and even your face, your skin, your eyes! Some day, I shall sit and talk to you about it all."

He then asked me to pull out a piece of paper and a pen. "Write down your prescription," he said.

I opened my mouth to ask how I could write my own prescription, but decided against voicing the question. After all, nothing in this session was going quite conventionally.

The prescription Vaidya Sharma dictated to me read as follows:

- Give yourself a warm sesame-oil full-body massage before your daily bath.
- Drink a cup of warm water every half hour.
- Make generous use of coarsely pounded coriander seeds in cooking.
- Eat a spoonful of rose-petal preserve at noon.
- Practice twenty minutes of quiet reflection every morning and evening.

I hesitated, then asked, "And the medicines?" He smiled. "My dear girl, your pulse tells me you are blessed with very strong immunity. I feel certain that my prescription will heal your infection quite easily. But to make sure you don't encounter these minor illnesses, use the medicines that are sitting on your spice rack, and those that are waiting inside your heart."

The good vaidya's words kindled in me a keen curiosity about Ayurveda. How I wished he would take the day off and talk to me about his methods, but his next patient was already at the door. I decided that my next-best source of information on this system of healing would be a good book. So off I went to the nearest public library, and fished out all the books on alternative healing that I could find.

I soon noticed a pattern: in most books, Ayurveda was sandwiched between aromatherapy and Chinese herbalism and defined as "a 5,000-year-old healing system from India that believes all human beings are combinations of three *doshas* — *vata*, *pitta*, and *kapha* — whose harmonious functioning is the key to good health." The dosha charts looked like this:

VATA: thin build, dry skin, rough nails, restless movements, volatile nature

PITTA: strong pulse, hot urine, reddish skin, loud voice, exaggerated emotions

KAPHA: strong build, soft skin, thick and greasy hair, slow digestion, relaxed nature

My meeting with Vaidya Sharma had led me to expect something different — something simpler. These unfamiliar terms jarred. Anyway, I attempted a What's-Your-Dosha quiz from one of the books. Yes, I was prone to rashes but, no, I didn't love hot weather. Yes, I was generally calm but, no, I didn't suffer frequent coughs and colds. So what did that make me? A jumbled mix of vata, pitta, and kapha. And armed with this extremely helpful information about myself, what was I supposed to do? I was clueless. It was time to see Vaidya Sharma again.

He heard me out, then shook his head. "Ah, yes, the doshas. It is true that you could call them the keystone of Ayurvedic healing. But unfortunately, in these impatient times, learning about the doshas has become a shortcut to understanding Ayurveda. I find that people quickly identify themselves as certain dosha types, then start treating their problems according to fixed dosha-balancing charts. But that is as unfair as watching the first few scenes of a film to write a complete review. Ayurveda is much more than the doshas, just as psychology is much more than Freud. That is why I don't introduce people to the doshas right away; I urge them to live their lives the Ayurveda way."

And what, I queried, was the Ayurveda way? "Learning how intimately your body and mind are connected, knowing what will make them work in harmony, and doing what you can to create that harmony. That is all there is to it."

With those words, Vaidya Sharma invited me to dip my toes into the Ayurvedic ocean. For the next fourteen years, I plumbed its fascinating depths. Today, I emerge — refreshed, rejuvenated, and ready to share with you the golden nuggets I found.

ayurveda: fascinating facts

1. How old is Ayurveda? No one really knows, but perhaps it is the oldest system of healing in the world. The Rig-Veda, India's oldest philosophical text, describes Ayurvedic theory in great detail in its verses; it was written somewhere between 4500 and 1600 B.C.

2. Ayurvedic theory in its entirety was recorded as an *upveda* (subtext) of the Yajur-Veda, one of the four ancient philosophical texts (Rig-Veda, Sama-Veda, Atharva-Veda, and Yajur-Veda) of India. It was authored sometime between 3000 and 2000 B.C. In keeping with the vedic tradition, the Ayurvedic text is written in verse form and is not the original work of any one person. Instead, it is the codification of health traditions passed down orally over the centuries.

3. How did Ayurveda originate? As ill-health grew in the ancient world, the sages of that time became concerned. To seek a deep understanding of human health and well-being, they held a convocation. Their chief, Sage Bharadwaj, sought the answers while the rest of the group sat deep in meditation. Together, the synergy of these great minds created a sublime moment of revelation that Sage Bharadwaj recognized as the very essence of Ayurveda. This is the

story of Ayurveda as recorded in the ancient vedic texts.

4. Legend apart, it is Sage Charaka who is widely credited as being Ayurveda's founding father. He is said to have been the world's first physician to describe multiple sclerosis, Alzheimer's disease, myasthenia gravis, Parkinson's disease, and many other well-known conditions.

5. Sage Susruta, said to be the world's first surgeon, is credited as being one of Ayurveda's principal healers along with Charaka. He described the month-by-month development of the fetus in the womb. His knowledge was corroborated many centuries later by modern science using state-of-the-art diagnostic instruments. For instance, Susruta says, "During the third month of pregnancy, all the sense organs and all the limbs emerge simultaneously. When the sense organs manifest and the latent mind activates, there is a throbbing sensation in the heart." Modern science now knows this is true.

---

CHAPTER 1

ayurveda is a verb

Aristotle: To be is to do.
Voltaire: To do is to be.
Frank Sinatra: Doobedoobedoobedoo

Nathaniel Hawthorne once wrote, "Happiness is a butterfly which, when pursued, is always just beyond your grasp, but which, if you will sit down quietly, may alight upon you."

Beautiful words.

But if an Ayurvedic healer were to substitute "health" for "happiness" here, I am certain he would put it like this: "Health is NOT a butterfly that will come and sit on your shoulder quietly. But give it a good chase, and you will have it in your grasp."

This, to me, is the sum and substance of Ayurveda. It sees good health not as an elusive lifelong quest, but as a duty you have to yourself every living moment.

Remember the unusual prescription Vaidya Sharma gave me (see introduction)? Let's look at it once more, this time with some of the words in bold print:

- **Give** yourself a warm sesame-oil massage before your daily bath.
- **Drink** a cup of warm water every half hour.
- **Make** generous use of coarsely pounded coriander seeds in cooking.
- **Eat** a spoonful of rose-petal preserve at noon.
- **Practice** twenty minutes of quiet reflection every morning and evening.

See? Each of the words highlighted is a verb.

That is why, although Ayurveda is rightly listed in the dictionary as a noun, I call it a verb. And that is why this book will tell you not only what Ayurveda can do for you, but how *you* can do Ayurveda.

So what exactly does the practice of Ayurveda ask you to do? Perform your *dharma* (religious duty), pursue *artha* (wealth and security), seek *kama* (pleasure), and strive for *moksha* (pursuit of liberation from earthly miseries) — the four efforts toward happiness as described in Hindu philosophy? Or reset your consciousness in order to drink from the fountain of eternal youth? Or contemplate the deeper reality of life while standing on your head?

Happily, the answer is "None of the above."

"Doing" Ayurveda does not require conquering complicated Sanskrit terms, memorizing mantras, mastering body contortions, or struggling with religious beliefs. It requires nothing except that you commit your time and energy to your own supreme well-being. What's more, it asks that you do this in as relaxed a manner as you like, step by baby step — a simple, friendly, and — yes — fun way to be 100 percent healthy!

In concrete terms, to "do" Ayurveda is to make healthy choices in daily life. These choices can be as simple as choosing fresh fruit over a donut, choosing a health magazine over a horror novel, choosing to sleep instead of watching a late-night film. I promise this is what Ayurveda is really about, even though you might have heard or read differently before picking up this book.

Because Ayurveda is about lifestyle, it follows that the most important element in following its principles is . . . you! From this moment onward, think of physicians as mere guides in your journey toward perfect health. Resolve to slowly wean yourself from your dependence on them. Revel in the heady knowledge that you can go the distance alone. Respect your own potential to heal and be whole, such self-respect is the essence of Ayurveda.

The Ayurvedic route to great health involves two simple steps:

1. Doing less;
2. Being more.

Before you set out toward your destination, keep one thing in mind: this is going to be a journey with a difference.

Here, one step doesn't follow the other; you take both simultaneously.

doing less, being more

Picture this: You have just emerged from a meeting with the boss, and for the next two hours you worry about the furrow on her brow, the grimace at the corner of her lips, the tone of her voice. Determined to win her smile by the end of the day, you immerse yourself in a sea of files. In doing this, you ignore your dry throat, your stale breath, your aching eyes, your strained neck, your throbbing wrist, your parched skin, and your stretched nerves. Later, at home, it's the spouse, kids, and dogs waiting for you to give them time, attention, and dinner.

All the time, in every way possible, other people are deciding the course of our actions. We are listening to them so hard, trying so desperately to please them, that we can no longer listen to ourselves. In "doing" all the time, we forget to just "be."

Ironically, over time, the more we "do," the less we achieve. All that effort takes its toll on our physical, mental, and emotional health. It disconnects us from our deeper needs, leaving us empty and dull. In rural India we have a saying: "If you keep drawing from it, even the deepest well will dry up one day." That is just what eventually happens; we dry up.

Now imagine a different, more pleasant scenario. You come to work determined to win your own smile at the end of the day. That is, you remember to log off your computer, take a short walk, drink a glass of water, and moisturize your skin every thirty minutes. Instead of "grabbing" an indifferent lunch, you bring fresh fruit, yogurt, and a whole-grain sandwich from home. You don't take coffee breaks, you take exercise breaks.

Just one day of treating yourself well is sure to set off a chain of happy events. You return to your desk humming after your short break, and suddenly the solution to a niggling little problem pops into your head. Even if nothing so dramatic happens, you find yourself being nice to your coworkers. Instead of the usual post-lunch slump, you feel a post-lunch kick. Back home, you want to make a good dinner instead of warming yesterday's meal.

In treating yourself well for a day, you achieved both doing less and being more. In the literal sense, you still "did" things; you did not sit idle. But what you did was gloriously different from what you had been doing for so long. You let yourself slow down instead of driving yourself hard. You did not misuse your body and you did not pressure your mind. You began the process of healing.

You lived Ayurveda today.

being more, bite by healthful bite

Surprising, isn't it, that a system of healing so ancient should seem so completely commonsense and user-friendly? It is, it is! What's more, the Ayurvedic love of harmony also extends to how you progress. The vaidya will always tell you that trying too hard to change old habits is in itself an enemy of harmony; it creates stress, and stress is the enemy of health. Let me tell you an interesting Indian folk tale that will bring home this point very nicely.

Before setting out to till the soil in her fields, a village woman called to her daughter: "Listen carefully, child. I shall return in the afternoon, so you can go out and play with your friends until then. But before you leave, I want you to sweep and mop the floors, make the beds, prepare bread, cook the lentils, clean the dishes, milk the cows, and fetch water from the well."

Overwhelmed by this torrent of instructions, the little girl could bring herself to do nothing but sit and weep. Just then, her father emerged from his morning prayer. When he heard the reason for his daughter's tears, he said, "I wish I could help you with your chores, little one. But I have to clean out the pigsty and chop a heap of wood. Don't worry, though. I'll make your job easy. Here: take this broom and start by sweeping the floor."

The girl set to work. When she had swept the floor, her father handed her the mop. After she was through mopping, he told her to go make the beds. And so on, step-by-step, until all her work was done before lunchtime.

"There, was that so hard?" inquired the father, his eyes twinkling. The girl shook her head happily and went out to play with her friends.

The moral of the story: Attack your goal of great health in bite-sized chunks, and you'll get there without overstepping your comfort zone. Don't kill yourself to live better!

awaken the doctor within you

Slowly, your new habit of doing less and being more will yield an excellent side benefit: you will be able to hear yourself better. (The great thing about Ayurveda is that its treatments always yield side benefits, not side effects.)

I will illustrate this notion of "hearing yourself better" by recounting an interesting incident. We were driving from Colorado to California on a family vacation, and I was quizzing my son on world geography. The FM radio station played softly in the background. Suddenly, my husband switched off the radio and said, "Shhh! I can hear a sound in the car."

"What sound?" I asked, after straining to hear it. All I could hear was the steady purr of the engine.

"There is a "clink" sound somewhere — and it comes about every thirty seconds," he insisted. I listened again — and couldn't catch any clinking. "Much ado about nothing," I muttered. But by this time, my husband was already pulling over.

Minutes later, he had his finger on the problem. "See this? The bearings on this wheel have worn off," he pointed out triumphantly. "We need to have them replaced as soon as we hit the next big town."

See what I'm getting at? My husband could catch the faint "clink" because he knew the normal sounds of his car intimately. Just like that, you can catch the off-key signals of your body when you learn to be in tune with it. As a result, if and when a tune-up is needed, you will not need to wait for a doctor to diagnose where the discordant note is coming from.

Speaking of doctors, another occasion comes to mind. Under attack from a particularly bad flu while reporting on television for the general election in India, I succumbed to the urge for quick relief and went to the nearest doctor I could find. He asked me to describe my symptoms, and I said, "My nose is completely blocked. My eyebrows and cheeks hurt. I think I have maxillo-facial sinusitis."

The doctor couldn't hide his astonishment. Then he pulled himself together and said, "Don't talk like a book." He proceeded to make the same diagnosis in pointedly medical terms, and wrote a prescription for some strong antibiotics (which blocked my nose even more thoroughly, but that is another story).

At first it struck me as strange that the doctor reacted negatively to my self-diagnosis. It was as if he found it absurd that a layperson should know the term "maxillo-facial sinusitis." But thinking back, I realize that the doctor's attitude was no mystery. Doctors are conditioned to see most of their patients as clueless people desperately seeking remedies. And they are justified in that assumption, because that is exactly what happens in most cases; we don't understand our maladies because we don't even try.

Try — and you will know. According to Ayurvedic principles, that's the way nature intended it.

To those of us who have been brought up to trust no one but the doctor, the pharmacist, and the medicines — and that covers most of us, I guess — this new idea of consulting ourselves can seem unrealistic and unconvincing at first. Therefore, I suggest that we examine this Ayurvedic belief system from the root upward.

the importance of action

Ayurvedic healers believe that you are not a mortal package of bone, muscle, and blood, but a part of the universe itself. They are convinced that you can be as rhythmic as the seasons, as powerful as any star, as ageless as time — because they believe that you are made up of the same dynamic elements that compose the cosmos. That is why they respect and trust you deeply.

Thousands of years ago, when Ayurveda was in its formative years, its sages had no microscopes, scalpels, or medical texts. The earth was their laboratory, and the wondrous universe their subject. While today it is nearly impossible for us to think of human biology without using terms like "organs," "tissues," and "genes," back then none of this vocabulary existed. Therefore, the sages slowly made their own connections and noted their own findings — using no other reference than life as they saw it.

I wonder when and how the idea first emerged that human beings were one with their universe, but emerge it did. Sometime during those long-gone centuries, the sages made the fascinating observation that the fire that burned in volcanoes also burned inside the human belly; the earth that bore life was also a constituent element of human physiology; and the boundless space all around was a vital part of the human body and mind.

From these basic observations flowed a series of conclusions: If human beings were indeed compact forms of the universe itself, then all the laws that governed the universe also governed them. This meant that the same unseen natural intelligence that controlled the rhythm of the seasons also regulated human digestion, respiration, circulation, and reproduction. And the intelligence that told a seed to send forth a giant tree also taught a broken bone to heal itself.

And yet, in spite of this supreme intelligence, disease struck. Men and women fell violently ill — or simply aged and died. The sages never stopped questioning why. Then they unlocked another important secret: the "intelligence" we possess has a "flow" that can be interrupted. They called this flow *prana*, or vital life force.

Impurities, imbalances, immoderation — one by one the enemies of flow emerged. What the sages now needed was to find the friend who could restore the flow of natural intelligence, thus defeating disease. Again and again, their attention was drawn to one and only one person: the sufferer himself. This was the person, Ayurvedic healers reasoned, who played host to both the intelligence and the interruption of flow.

Yes! The sick knew exactly where their discomfort lay. They alone could tell what made them feel better.

Who better qualified than the suffering, the healers reasoned, to be the friends they were searching for?

In other words, the answer to each human disease and disorder lay within the individual human being.

When Vaidya Divakar Sharma first explained this theory to me, I was skeptical. After all, I argued, how can I be a better doctor to myself than an actual, medical-degree-holding doctor who knows the human body inside and out? The vaidya calmly pointed out that a doctor does know the human body better, but he can never know my body better than me.

That made perfect sense. And, to bring this chapter full circle, it convinces me that Ayurveda is, above everything else, a verb.

ayurveda spells health
b-a-l-a-n-c-e

*The same stream of life that runs through my veins night
and day runs through the world and dances in rhythmic
measures. It is the same life that is rocked in the ocean-cradle
of birth and of death, in ebb and in flow.*

— Rabindranath Tagore

Imagine a tripod with one leg missing. Can you see it
standing straight? According to Ayurveda, just as a tripod cannot stand on two legs, you cannot be in perfect
health if any one of these three elements is not in balance:

- body
- mind
- soul

We experience the truth of this statement all the
time: a bad day at work may trigger bodily aches and

13

pains; a toothache could result in depression; the loss of a loved one can lead to a stroke.

Yet practitioners of modern medicine insist on addressing body and mind as separate entities; a heart specialist asks you about your cholesterol level, not about your love life. As a consequence, you have different doctors for different parts: bone specialists, urologists, cardiologists, therapists.

An Ayurvedic physician, however, is always a vaidya. Period. A vaidya is trained to treat you as a whole being, complete with your bone, muscle, kidneys, skin type, likes and dislikes, habits, thoughts, and feelings. And, interestingly, whatever your symptom and however chronic your problem, the diagnosis is always the same: imbalance. This imbalance can be in your physiology, your psychology, or your very spirit. But an imbalance it always is.

So, with apologies to John Keats, I would sum up the Ayurvedic definition of health thus: "Balance is health, and health balance: that is all ye know on earth and all ye need ever know."

Now, balance may seem to be an abstract thing. So is it possible to set about achieving it the way you would, say, a monthly sales goal? Or does it mean straying into the realm of heart, soul, and such abstract things?

The answer lies somewhere in between. That is because part of good health can be quantified (blood-pressure readings, cholesterol count, heart rate), but an equal part of it can only be judged by quality (calm, optimism, equanimity).

Therefore, I suggest that you start by thinking of your quest for balance as an endeavor to learn an art. I like to think of it as working with clay; healing and making pottery echo each other beautifully.

Have you ever seen a master potter at work? How magically the potter, with delicate fingers and a light touch, turns shapeless clay into a perfect, symmetrical teapot in seconds. But if you have ever tried your hand at pottery, you know what those fingers are doing while the fragile clay spins furiously on the wheel. In those few seconds, they are shaping, steadying, lifting, pressing, pulling, centering, dimpling, raising, and leveling the clay.

I got a firsthand idea of the master potter's job three years ago at a pottery workshop, where I tried my hand at "throwing" a pot. Having watched the instructor turn out two perfect pots in two minutes, I felt that it would be child's play. How mistaken I was! I tried to make a pot six times, but each time — at the crucial shaping stage when I slowly lifted the neck — the clay would spin out of control and break into a miserable, shapeless lump. It was terribly frustrating.

The instructor knew exactly where I was going wrong. "Try to balance your pot," he said. "When you cup that clay between your palms, feel for the slightest lump and the faintest bump. Any protrusion or dent that manages to hide in those tender walls will cause them to lose balance, and the weakest spot will tear."

Those words exactly reflect the Ayurvedic view of perfect health. In Ayurvedic terms, all illness begins with the tiniest chink or dent in the human vessel. That is why I invite you to put yourself in the role of a potter in love with the clay of your being. Take your body, your thoughts, and your emotions as the malleable clay spinning on the wheel of time, and mold them into a perfectly balanced work of art: a vessel free of lumps, bumps, and dents. Thus balanced, you will be a living embodiment of the Ayurvedic word for "healthy": *swastha*. (*swa:* self, *stha:* established/steady — "established in the self").

How does it feel to be balanced? I am sure you have known that feeling on days when you sing while cooking breakfast, lavish someone with compliments, or pirouette around the house for no reason at all. In those rare moments, without even realizing it, you have achieved perfect balance among the following elements:

- your own body, mind, and heart;
- yourself and other people;
- yourself and your surroundings.

For many of us, such moments of complete balance are but pleasant interludes in the tense drama of life. But once you understand and follow Ayurveda, it need not be this way. You can make sure that imbalance, not balance, is the exception in your life. What's more, with Ayurveda as your road map, you can take the scenic route to balance.

And now, let's get down to the brass tacks of the journey. What's the first thing you do before you start on a coast-to-coast trip? You tune in to weather and road conditions, check for possible delays, and fix your vehicle for the trip. Similarly, before you set out to re-create balance in your own being, you need to figure out where the lumps and bumps lie.

identifying your imbalances

According to the Ayurvedic approach, there are two key causes of imbalance:

1. external factors (for example, change of season, pollution, and infection);
2. internal causes (chiefly the accumulation of toxic matter inside us).

The external enemies of balance find it easy to gatecrash when our inner defenses are down. Also, they are more or less beyond our control. The internal enemy — toxic pileup — is one we can combat and defeat. Therefore, our focus should be on cleaning out these toxins. What exactly are these toxins and how do they affect us?

Toxins are easy to understand if you look at the human body as a network of channels; think of them as specialized courier services that receive and deliver packages. Men have thirteen such channels — called *shrotas* in Ayurveda — while women have fifteen, including the reproductive channels.

Package	Couriers
Air	heart, lungs, abdomen
Food	stomach, intestines
Water	palate, pancreas, skin, kidneys, bladder
Plasma	heart, blood vessels, lymphatic system
Blood	liver, spleen, blood vessels, arteries, capillaries
Muscle nutrients	ligaments, tendons, skin
Fat	fatty tissue, arteries
Bone nutrients	teeth, hips, joints
Bone marrow	marrow, nerve tissue
Ovum/sperm	testes, ovaries
Urine	kidneys, bladder
Feces	colon, rectum
Sweat	fatty tissue, hair follicles
Menses	uterus (only in women)
Milk	breasts (only in women)

Similarly, the mind and the heart are couriers of thought and emotion.

Try to imagine a traffic jam in any one department, and you can see how easy it is to create chaos and breakdown in the entire channel network. Take the example of blood pooling in the veins of the lower foot — something that happens to many people. To begin with, poor circulation results in poor distribution of nutrients across the cells and tissues. It also reduces the flow of oxygen to and from the body, causing irregular heartbeat, dizziness, and fatigue. The feet swell up and the blood can form clots. In serious cases a clot can travel to the lungs, becoming a potentially fatal pulmonary embolism.

In fact, the root of most minor and major illnesses is some kind of blockage: a tooth pocket filled with plaque, mucus-choked sinuses, accumulated fat, a stone blocking the gall bladder, a clogged artery.

At the stage when toxins are still building up, we sense discomfort, pain, and restlessness. When the jam becomes crippling, we give the resulting disease a name: cystitis, arthritis, diabetes, depression, heart disease, cancer.

Until I began studying Ayurveda, I didn't realize how easy it is to collect toxins on an average day without even trying. My daily toxin pile accumulates from small acts of neglect: eating a late dinner, omitting to moisturize my skin, breathing shallowly all day, sitting hunched for hours over my computer, hurting over an insensitive comment.

On a rushed day, I go on my toxin-collecting spree more systematically. I work late into the night, depriving my body and mind of the rest they need. I wake up irritable and groggy, with little appetite for breakfast. Whatever appetite I have, I douse with three continuous cups of coffee. I go to work and plunge straightaway into the waiting files. I make careless mistakes, then simmer when they're pointed out. Just before a crucial meeting, I find I have gone completely blank. How do these acts of neglect translate into actual physical toxins? They generate such substances as acid, bile, cholesterol, and adrenaline. In moderate amounts, these are essential to life. But produced in excess, they overwhelm the body, compromising its ability to perform the routine functions of metabolism and digestion normally.

Thus burdened on the home front, the body finds it increasingly difficult to keep away the enemies straining at its barriers — smoke, dust, nitrates, pesticides — and the agents of disease begin to stroll in. In this stage of weakened immunity, the body becomes what vaidyas call a *beej-bhoomi*, or "breeding ground" (*beej* means "seed," and *bhoomi* is Sanskrit for "earth"), for disease to take root. It is a seedbed for disease to thrive in, fed with the manure of toxins by a self-destructive gardener. Not a pretty image, but alas true.

In Ayurveda, these toxins are called *ama* (pronounced "aa-ma"). This deceptively sweet-sounding Sanskrit word literally means "unripe, immature, undigested." All undigested, toxic matter inside you is ama — whether in the form of food, bile, acid, or negative thoughts.

ama up close

Because the Ayurvedic perspective encompasses the total picture, it takes into account toxins that germinate in both body and mind. Ama, therefore, is both physical and mental. If ignored for too long, it can even seep into the soul.

Physical Ama

Ama in the body almost always begins with ineffi-cient digestion. When your lifestyle is at odds with the needs of your constitution — you skip meals, eat foods that are not right for you, and eat at the wrong time — your body's vital digestive fire, which vaidyas call *jatharagni,* dims. As a result, food fails to be totally digested and properly absorbed.

Undigested food, or ama, sits in the stomach and putrefies, releasing toxic chemicals. Slowly, it clogs the intestines and prevents the colon from assimilating nutri-ents from digested food.

In Ayurveda, this kind of ama is described as a sticky, white, foul-smelling substance that blocks arteries and capillaries. It jams the tissues and cells of the body. This, in turn, inhibits the free flow of water, blood, wastes, nutrients, and air in the system. If neglected, ama spreads and lodges in the tiniest circulatory channels of your body, causing a plethora of symptoms ranging from unease and bloating to heaviness and pain.

These symptoms are your body's SOS signals, telling you that ama has weakened your innate capacity to heal yourself. Your body is asking you for help.

Why not help your body before it is forced to ask for assistance? It's easy to do. From time to time, check for ama buildup by asking yourself some basic questions:

- Is my breathing slow and steady, deep and unre-stricted?

- Is my appetite keen?
- Do I experience thirst at regular intervals?
- Is my waste (urine, stool, sweat) output normal? (Healthy urine is light-colored and odor-free, occurring without obstruction or urgency; healthy stool occurs once or twice a day, floats in water, and does not smell foul; sweat should be free of strong odor— and not be either profuse or insufficient.)
- Are my five senses (sight, hearing, taste, touch, and smell) performing well?
- Is my skin lustrous and supple?
- Am I generally free of ulcers, lumps, and bumps?
- Do I feel active and energetic?
- Is my breath fresh and are my teeth strong?
- Are my joints well-lubricated and healthy?
- Is my sexual urge normal?
- Do I sleep well?

Do you notice the common thread that runs through these seemingly diverse questions? That thread is blockage. You're checking for obstruction in all areas of your body — from hunger and vision to elimination and energy. Your answers should give you a fair idea of your ama levels while also pinpointing the trouble spots. I strongly recommend paying attention to the clues you receive from this test. Small discomforts and complaints — whether slight trouble focusing on faraway objects or a recurrent muscle twitch — indicate that disorder is still at an elementary stage and can be turned around with positive effort.

One obvious sign of ama in your system is a coated,

"furry" tongue. That is why vaidyas ask you to open your mouth and stick out your tongue; the amount and color of coating on your tongue gives them vital information about the extent to which ama has accumulated in your system.

Mental and Emotional Ama

Though you cannot see it, you can sense non-physiological ama. You can feel it in the little irritations and anxieties that pile up during your day. Slowly, these negative thoughts and energies multiply, leading to bigger problems such as insomnia and depression.

The loss of a loved one, tension at work, divorce — these are the big ama generators. The mind cannot easily process them and the heart cannot easily "digest" them. A pang of jealousy or a creative block will make a small but significant contribution to your reservoir of emotional ama.

Here is a quick mental-ama assessment test. Before you take it, a word of advice: Answer these questions when you are in a relaxed frame of mind so that you can analyze your responses without being filled with guilt or alarm. If you do find yourself being swamped by those feelings, remember two things:

1. The purpose here is not to chide yourself; it is to read your slate as it is, then decide how to wipe off the smudged portions and write a new script on it. Just like a slow, steady hand prints neat letters, a slow and relaxed approach to rewriting your health will always work best.

2. A good gardener knows why leaves develop brown patches; there is a problem at the root

level. Similarly, this little quiz could guide you to the root of your own emotional behavior. And when you start from the depths, there's only one way things can go: upward.

Here are the questions that will help you assess your level of mental ama:

- Am I happy at work?
- Do I have a stable family life and a strong support system?
- Am I happy with my partner?
- Do I have a strong relationship with my co-workers and friends?
- Is my ability to rest — both physically and mentally — adequate?
- Do I handle difficult situations calmly?
- Do I have enough leisure time and do I make positive use of it?
- Do I usually feel calm inside?

You may not have realized it, but this test also gave you a complete self-exam; you actually checked out how your bodily and mental channels are performing. The more often you do this quick check, the closer you will come to knowing your body and mind.

catching ama early

The tyranny of stressful living makes it impossible to resist assault from ama. But we can do the next best thing: slow it down and flush it out regularly.

This is where your actions count; by choosing fresh fruit over a sugar-laden donut and by giving your lunch priority over that pending file, you can refuse to let ama accumulate in your body. Also, by drinking plenty of water and getting adequate exercise, you can eliminate ama from your body at regular intervals. The sweeping action of water ferries toxins to their exit points, keeping the channels clear. I think of it as making sure a kitchen sink always drains well instead of trying to unclog a choked drain. Similarly, exercise improves circulation, thus helping the body flush out toxins faster.

A good strategy for keeping physical ama in check is to reassign the roles played by your mind and your senses. It is easy and habitual to let your senses control your actions. For instance, when you reach out for onion rings in spite of your ulcer, you are ignoring the advice of your mind. But if you give the reins to your mind, you will pass over those onion rings and reach for a glass of water instead.

Tackling ama of the mind and heart requires a different approach. Most of our abstract ama is generated when we pull the mind away from the realm of tranquillity where it naturally wants to go. We chase ephemeral material objects instead of realizing and fulfilling our own deeper needs. In the bargain, all we really get is a heart full of sorrow and a mind empty of joy.

It is, therefore, as important to nourish the mind as it is to feed the body. Reading an uplifting book with your spouse, taking a sixty-second mental vacation when you're tired, giving more freely to others — these small actions work like vitamins and minerals in your psyche, strengthening and toning it.

While these general guidelines work well for everyone, regardless of gender or nationality, each of us is unique. Therefore, your strategy for achieving freedom from ama should be devised in accordance with your own nature.

how toxins become disease

All disease, according to Ayurvedic thought, progresses in six steady steps:

1. *Sanchaya:* the earliest stage of disease. At this point, toxic ama starts to accumulate, hampering free circulation of the vital energies.
2. *Prakopa:* the disease enters its second phase, in which the doshas are aggravated or excited, causing further channel blockage.
3. *Prasara:* the accumulated ama moves from the digestive tract into other organs of the body, impairing the doshas and their energies even further.
4. *Sthanasamsarya:* the moving ama settles in a localized area.
5. *Vyakti:* the disease manifests itself and the sufferer feels its symptoms.
6. *Bheda:* untreated or neglected, the disease acquires chronic — sometimes untreatable — dimensions.

how ayurvedic healing works

He has the healing touch — that magnetic thing
which defies explanation or analysis.

— Sir Arthur Conan Doyle

Have you ever sought a doctor's appointment just because you're feeling "sort of funny"?

Has your doctor ever outlined a new food plan for you just by looking at your tongue?

Have you ever returned from seeing your doctor with the advice "take a walk in the moonlight" on your prescription?

The answer to all the above questions can be "Yes" if your doctor is an Ayurvedic one — that is, a vaidya.

meet the vaidya

A vaidya does not go to Harvard, of course. A vaidya does not wear a white coat, or even a blue one. A vaidya does not pull out a thermometer or a stethoscope, and doesn't write you prescriptions for drugs.

So what kind of a doctor is this vaidya?

A vaidya is a fully trained holistic physician. To become a vaidya, a person studies eight diverse branches of medicine for many laborious years. These fields of study are called:

1. *Kaya Chikitsa:* internal medicine
2. *Bal Chikitsa:* pediatrics
3. *Graha Chikitsa:* psychiatry
4. *Shalakya Tantra:* eye, ear, nose, and throat treatment
5. *Shalya Tantra:* surgery
6. *Agad Tantra:* toxicology
7. *Rasayan Tantra:* geriatrics (the study of old age and rejuvenation)
8. *Vajikarana Tantra:* aphrodisiacs and fertility

Vaidyas have studied these same branches of medicine for 1,500 years. The difference between then and now is that Ayurvedic physicians today also learn about human anatomy, nutrition, and other aspects of modern medicine. Thus, they combine ancient wisdom with cutting-edge medical knowledge.

In India, becoming a vaidya requires six years of study in an Ayurvedic college or university. In addition to academic education, many vaidyas have acquired their knowledge of Ayurveda from their families.

The story goes that when the Moguls invaded India, they burned down the entire library of Ayurvedic books at the prestigious Nalanda University in eastern India. To compensate for that loss, the vaidyas of that time committed all of Ayurvedic knowledge to memory and passed it on to their sons. These sons — now a select few vaidyas — received Ayurveda in their very genes. Along with their formal training, the invaluable experience of learning from and working with their fathers made them the best among healers. I have the privilege of working with one of them — Vaidya Ramakant Mishra, whose ancestors were physicians to the kings of India.

the ayurvedic definition of a healer

Let us look further at the difference between the Western and Ayurvedic approaches to healing. In the Western world, a healer is generally the doctor or physician who treats you. A visit to the Western physician is usually a formal affair. The well-appointed clinics, state-of-the-art diagnostic tools, and often polite-but-detached advice (perhaps out of fear of lawsuits?) all play their role in giving the modern physician the image of an automobile mechanic. To be fair, not all Western physicians are aloof or detached, but all too often this is the ambiance of Western medical treatment.

Writer Anatole Broyard once said, "A doctor, like a writer, must have a voice of his own — something that conveys the timbre, the rhythm, the diction, and the music of his humanity that compensates us for all the speechless machines." To my mind, Broyard's words draw a beautiful picture of the Ayurvedic physician. Because a vaidya perceives the patient as an individual with unique characteristics and unique problems, Ayurvedic methods of healing resonate with "the music of humanity."

In India, vaidyas have always enjoyed a high status. In my mother's village, the local *vaidyaji* (*ji* is a suffix added as a mark of respect) was lavished with tokens of patients' gratitude. My mother tells me that he even played the role of general counselor on matters such as marriage, buying and selling property, and forecasting the weather.

This reverence dates back to a time when the vaidya was regarded as not only a physician but also a sage. Knowledge of healing was said to come directly to the vaidya by divine revelation. The erstwhile kings of India had their own personal physicians, who not only kept the royal family in good health but also performed religious rites. The old treatises say that a vaidya must possess enough knowledge, training, and experience to bring the patient balance in body, mind, and soul. The leading light of Ayurveda, Sage Charaka, urges the vaidya to "enter the body of a patient with the lamp of knowledge and understanding."

other elements of ayurvedic healing

In addition to the vaidya, there are three other — and no less important — components of the Ayurvedic healing process.

The Medicine

Ayurvedic pharmacology is called *dravyaguna* (*dravya* means "healing ingredient"; *guna* means "quality"). Ayurvedic medicines are prepared from plants without isolating their active ingredients. Thus, Ayurvedic drugs retain their natural synergy and are largely free of side effects.

Sage Charaka identified 350 species of healing plants, then divided them into fifty groups based on the actions — preventive or curative — of the medicines that could be extracted from them. These medicines included tonics for the heart, analgesics, anti-inflammatories, purgatives, fertility enhancers, bone-setting compounds, and diuretics. In his compendium on healing, the *Charaka Samhita*, he describes a good medicine as being readily available, easy to administer, safe, and effective. The *Samhita* also gives precise instructions on when and how to harvest a certain healing herb or plant, including the time of day. This is because Ayurvedic healers believe that everything in nature — including plants — has a biological rhythm that determines when it is at its most effective.

Because of the purity and potency of most Ayurvedic herbs, it is important not to self-administer them. Taken in the precise combination and amount recommended by a vaidya, however, most Ayurvedic herbal formulations are free of side effects.

Often a vaidya will prescribe a formulation that is less a drug than a food supplement. Prepared from precise blends of herbs and fruit, such formulations heal the body-mind as a whole. They strengthen the immune system, thus removing toxins and building up resistance to disease. Such formulations are given the status of a *rasayana* — something that supports the body's essential fluids, or *rasa;* specifically the blood and plasma.

The Patient

Ideally, one shouldn't reach the stage of being a "patient," the whole orientation of Ayurveda being toward prevention. But, of course, people do fall ill. That is why Ayurvedic texts dwell at length on the role of the person in the grip of a disorder. They instruct patients to describe their disease clearly, follow the physician's advice carefully, and maintain a positive attitude toward their illness.

It is also the patient's duty to work toward recognizing an imbalance before disease can take root. In real terms, this is how you would do it: Put down this book, and close your eyes if it helps you concentrate better. Now ask yourself if you are comfortable: is the room too hot or too cold for you? Are you snug in your clothes and shoes? Did you eat a good breakfast? How did you feel when you woke up this morning — did you spring out of bed or did you burrow deeper into the pillow to shut out the alarm clock? These seemingly trivial questions — and their answers — can often help you catch an imbalance early.

The Attendant

Usually a family member, friend, or nurse, the attendant forms a vital fourth dimension of the Ayurvedic healing process. The attendant should possess loyalty and love for the patient, accurate knowledge of the patient's disease, the skill to attend to the patient's needs, and the ability to keep the patient cheerful.

when should you see a vaidya?

The idea of seeing a doctor if you don't have a full-blown cold or fever can seem somewhat strange. It's not strange in the Ayurvedic scheme of things, however.

A vaidya is trained to catch disease at its very seed level. At that point, toxic ama is still at a stage when it can be flushed out easily through simple diet and lifestyle altera-tions. Think of it as pulling out a young weed; give it one light twist and it is out, root and all. Similarly, vaidyas like to weed out disease before it gets a chance to grow.

Therefore, you can see a vaidya even if your com-plaints are "minor" in nature — flatulence, general tired-ness, or simply not feeling your best. The vaidya will respect your complaint and give it the attention it deserves. You will be perceived as a sum of your body, mind, and spirit, not as a simple machine with an obvi-ous part in need of repair.

Once you develop an intuitive relationship with your own being, you can begin to develop a sense of your own subtle symptoms. With practice, it is possible to literally sniff an illness weeks before it can manifest itself just like a meteorologist can predict a weekend snowstorm on Monday morning.

I am reminded of an experience I had many years ago. Winter had just tiptoed into New Delhi, and the evenings were nippy. Yet that night I felt excessively thirsty. Not unwell — just very thirsty. When I poured myself a sixth glass of water, my grandmother said, "I think you are going to be unwell." Sure enough, the next morning my forehead was hot. I was laid up with viral fever for a week.

My grandmother's prediction might seem impressive, but I know that if a vaidya had seen me a week before I fell ill, he would have made the same prediction at that time. How would he have been able to do this? As Vaidya Divakar Sharma told me, every living moment the human body gives out clues about its health, and the vaidya is trained to detect the most minute ones.

how a vaidya sees you

Thousands of years ago, Sage Charaka set forth a comprehensive ten-point diagnostic checklist for vaidyas. Ayurvedic physicians study and follow that list to this day. Here is what Charaka asked vaidyas to check for:

1. *Prakriti:* the patient's basic constitution, which determines such factors as susceptibility to disease, digestive efficiency, work capacity, sleep requirement, and coping abilities.
2. *Vikriti:* the patient's current physical and psychological imbalances, studied against the background of his or her natural constitution.

3. *Sara:* the body components (skin and hair texture, complexion, luster of the eyes, and resonance of the voice).

4. *Samhanana:* the physical build (bone structure, height, length of joints, posture).

5. *Pramana:* the state of development of physical features, such as height and weight, in proportion to the patient's age.

6. *Satmya:* the patient's habits, especially those that have become second nature through repeated practice (for instance, an individual's adaptation to milk, cold weather, or job stress).

7. *Sattva:* the patient's mental makeup. The more positive the person's mental qualities, the faster and better the healing process. An action-oriented person will respond well to the correct remedy, while a sluggish person's disease can be stubborn and acute.

8. *Ahara Shakti:* the patient's appetite and digestive capacity, which are clues to the nature and extent of a disease.

9. *Vyayama Shakti:* the patient's capacity to exercise or work.

10. *Vaya:* the relationship between the patient's age and disease condition.

And to think that this comprehensive range of observations is made without the vaidya ever touching you! What's more, this is only the first stage in an Ayurvedic diagnosis. In fact, the ten stages mentioned here don't even cover the finer points that a vaidya notices. At this first stage, called *darshana,* or observation, the Ayurvedic physician is taking in not only your chief physical characteristics, but also such minute details as the thickness of your lips, the size of your tongue, and even the number of times you blink — all the while making pleasant small talk with you.

If the elaborate nature of this diagnosis makes you wonder, suffice it to say for now that every single one of these observations is like a nugget of gold to a vaidya. Your posture, your gait, and your smile speak volumes about your personality, your basic nature, and your current imbalances. That information, as you will see, is the bedrock upon which Ayurvedic healing rests.

The next stage in Ayurvedic diagnosis is *sparsha,* or touch. While a vaidya will also palpate your abdomen, the "touch" part of the diagnosis essentially begins with taking your pulse. From the moment the vaidya feels the first wave of the artery just beneath your wrist, lightning-quick signals from your body start being transmitted.

How does this happen? The Ayurvedic belief is that the circulatory channels — the arteries, veins, and capillaries — carry more than just vital nutrients; they also ferry vital information about your current state of health.

There is a reason why the vaidya always uses three fingers in pulse-diagnosis: each finger probes a specific aspect of your physiology. The first finger feels the energy of your body's motion-based functions (for example, respiration and circulation), the second finger perceives metabolic activity, and the third picks up signals about structural health (joints and muscles).

Pressing slightly harder, the vaidya gets a sense of how your deeper body channels (veins, capillaries, lymph) and tissues are doing. At this time, vaidyas can even pick up vital genetic information about you.

The final stage in an Ayurvedic diagnosis is *prashna*, or questioning. This stage differs from the ten-point diagnosis in stage one as the latter is based largely on observation and casual conversation while the former is structured with a more specific line of questioning. Like a Western physician, a vaidya will ask you questions. But a vaidya's line of questioning is very different. Unlike a Western physician, a vaidya does not ask, "When was the last time this happened?" "Where exactly do you feel it?" "How long has it been hurting?" and so on. Instead, a vaidya's questions are geared toward confirming the preliminary findings. Therefore, you can expect the vaidya to ask, "Have you been attending too many parties lately?" "Have you been suffering from constipation?" "Are you feeling overstressed these days?" Whereas a Western physician is likely to ask, "How long have you had this problem?" a vaidya is likely to ask, "Have you had this problem for the last two weeks?" The vaidya is able to assess the duration and extent to which a person has been suffering based on how much ama he senses in a person's system.

Fascinating, aren't they, the vaidya's subtle methods? Each time I pick up an Agatha Christie novel, ace sleuth Hercule Poirot reminds me of the vaidyas I have met over the years. Poirot was able to piece together the puzzle of a murdered woman using such seemingly meaningless clues as a broken mirror, a piece of blotting paper, and the remains of a fire in the grate!

restoring the balance

Not only does the vaidya cull information about you as a whole, but the line of treatment is also designed toward treating you as a whole. This is why the vaidya does not give you medicines that show results within twenty-four hours or administer shots to take care of your flu or phlegm. What the vaidya does is to offer you some simple, solid advice on how to live more health-fully. A consultation with a vaidya usually consists of guidelines on regulating your mealtimes, making changes in your diet, and getting a better quality of sleep. In addition, you might be advised to explore the tremendous healing powers of yoga, meditation, aro-matherapy, music therapy, and home-architecture ther-apy (called *Vastu* — an older cousin of feng shui). And, yes, a vaidya will give you some gentle herbal medication if that is appropriate.

Vaidyas like to start by talking about your diet. Their recommendations on good nutrition are often so simple that you might wonder if they are taking your disease seriously enough. But remember: the vaidya is trying to correct an imbalance. And most imbalances, according to Ayurvedic theory, originate when the digestion process is not functioning as it should.

We all know how it feels when work forces us to miss or delay a meal, or after we give in to our taste buds and indulge in a big chunk of cream pie. Those feelings — ranging from weakness to bloatedness — are our body's signals that the metabolic system is under stress. A vaidya doesn't even need to ask if you're feeling any of those things, instead perceiving your body's signals through observation and touch. Based on the strength of those signals, the vaidya will tell you which aspect of your food intake you need to improve: the quality, quantity, timing, or all of these.

Yes, vaidyas do make specific recommendations about what to eat and what to avoid. This can, understandably, worry some people. As Mark Twain said, "He had much experience of physicians, and said, 'The only way to keep your health is to eat what you don't want, drink what you don't like, and do what you'd rather not.'" Relax. A vaidya will give you a variety of ingredients to choose from. If the vaidya asks you to eat rutabagas and you don't relish them, just say so; there are other options.

Another word of advice: Don't take a vaidya's recommendations as absolutes. In my early days of trying Ayurvedic therapy, I went berserk trying to get exactly the amount of fennel and coriander in my diet that the vaidya had suggested. I soon realized, however, that Ayurveda is not about following lists. It is designed to awaken your body's own healing intelligence by giving it positive support. Therefore, as long as I was getting coriander in my diet and eating a regular breakfast, I was on the right track.

During a consultation with a vaidya, questions are bound to occur to you: "Why is cardamom good for me and not cloves? Why do I need to avoid ketchup? I wonder why he asked me to cut down on my workout — I thought working out was the best thing I could do for my health!" Don't be afraid to ask questions and seek clarification. Some vaidyas are good communicators; others might refrain from explaining the concepts of Ayurveda because they don't want to overwhelm you. But if you ask, they will willingly explain. Sometimes language can be a barrier, too; though a vaidya practicing in Europe or America will know basic English, an accent can be hard to understand at first.

This is where reading a good basic guide on Ayurveda will help you tremendously (see the resource section at the end of this book). Armed with some background knowledge, you'll be able to understand the reasoning behind much of what the vaidya says — and then you can ask more specific questions.

A session with a vaidya, then, is no doubt an interesting experience. But even more fascinating than the vaidya's methods are the principles on which the diagnosis is based. Can you imagine, for instance, that a vaidya taking your pulse is feeling the energies of fire, earth, water, air, and space coursing through your veins? Tantalizing, isn't it? Wait until you hear more — in the next chapter.

take your own pulse

Although pulse diagnosis is a specialized art, it can be rewarding to try to understand the rhythm of your own pulse from time to time. You can take your pulse anytime during the day. Your pulse will feel different at different times.

- If you're male, take the pulse on your right wrist.
- If you're a female, take the pulse on your left wrist.
- Use three fingers — the index, middle, and ring fingers — to press down on your pulse.
- Feel your pulse. How would you describe it? Light, rapid, slow, or jerky?

Your familiarity with the rhythm of your pulse can help you understand your current state of health, but a vaidya is the best person to help guide you on how to interpret your pulse-signals. With practice and guidance from your vaidya, you will be well equipped to regularly monitor your current state of health and, in turn, you will grow to know and understand the unique rhythms of your pulse-signals.

"elementary" ayurveda

Who in the world am I?
Ah! That's the great puzzle.

— Lewis Carroll

Before writing this chapter, I asked three people to answer a question: What image does the word "fire" conjure up for you?

The answers I got were:

- A burning forest.
- A firefighter in action.
- An erupting volcano.

While all of these are perfectly valid answers, my purpose in asking this question was to show you how differently a vaidya looks at an element of nature. To the vaidya, fire is the light in your eye, the heat that digests your food, the freckle on your face, the creative energy of your brain.

That is how the vaidya perceives each of the five elements of nature — earth, fire, air, water, and ether — in the context of its relationship to *you*. To the vaidya, these elements control every single activity within your being, from breathing and circulation to waste elimination and thinking. What's more, the vaidya believes that, just as our universe cannot exist without these elements inside it, you too cannot live without them. Quite simply, the person you call *you* is but a sum of the five elements of nature.

You might think that this is a fascinating, if somewhat overly romantic, way to look at life — at least until you study the theory a bit more deeply and realize how stunningly logical it is.

Throughout life, you have probably understood yourself through the perspective of modern biology: digestion is chemicals breaking down solid food matter, the blush on your cheeks is actually a rush of blood, and the sweat on your skin is the body's way of eliminating waste; hepatitis is a disease of the liver, and nephritis is a kidney disorder; heart attacks happen because cholesterol chokes the arteries.

Now, just for a while, look at yourself with a fresh pair of eyes. Forget the vocabulary of cells, tissues, and organs. Imagine yourself as an intense, bubbling cauldron of life — inside of which the five elements merge and flow. Imagine your aches, pains, and other health problems as being the result not of indisposed organs, but of the up-and-down swings of the five restless elements: earth (the Sanskrit word for earth is *prithvi*), fire (*agni*), water (*jal*), air (*vayu*), and ether (*akash*).

Let's take one element at a time.

First, think of all the fire inside you. What is hunger, but a burning flame that demands fuel? What is digestion, but the "burning up" of food to produce energy? Could "fire in the belly" be more than a metaphor? Envision the two bright dots in the pupils of your eyes as lit sparks. Touch the warmth of your rose-hued face as you come in from the snow. Feel the intensity of your words as they rise from your heart and form in your throat. The anger you sometimes feel is so close to fire; look at the metaphors we use to describe it: his cheeks burned, she simmered, my blood boiled. Yes, you are a creature of fire!

Next, turn your attention to earth. In this new perspective, earth is not just a planet that revolves around the sun, or solid physical matter with a core and crust. Think of it as the anchor of life — everything that gives support and structure to your being — from your spinal column to the ligaments that connect your muscles. Run your fingers through the earthy texture of your hair. Feel the rich loamy soil of your heart, where feelings of love and kindness grow and flourish.

Then, consider the prime mover of everything: the all-pervading air. Inhale deeply, and feel the warm current that flows in and out of your nostrils every living moment. What is it that powers and propels food, blood, waste, reproductive fluid, energy, and thought throughout your being? How do emotions — positive and negative — pollinate themselves across the soil of your heart? Who is the carrier of all these things but the mighty force of air? To the Ayurvedic healer, air is not a mixture of oxygen, nitrogen, and helium; it is prana, or life.

Water irrigates and lubricates. But inside the human body, water takes many forms. Every bead of moisture in you is water: the wetness of saliva in your mouth, the blood that courses through your veins, the tears that keep your eyes moist, the mucus that lines your nose, the gastric juices that process food, the fluid that keeps your joints supple, the ejaculate that generates life, and the protoplasm that fills every living cell.

Ether, or space, is an interesting element. On the face of it, you are a solid mass of cells and tissues firmly held together. But in reality, ether is everywhere; each cell in our body is separated by space. More obviously, space fills the cavities of the nose, ears, mouth, and genitals. But ether works on a much deeper level. It's the medium through which you can connect with your consciousness. In the cacophony of daily life, it is impossible to be aware of ether. But once you tune in to yourself, your mind's finest impulses travel through ether to seep into your consciousness — and that is the first step toward retuning the instrument of your being.

Now, can you ever again think of yourself as just another concoction of organs held together by bones and sewn inside a skin? But this new picture of yourself should also tell you something else: If you are a dynamo made from these diverse, restless elements, then you cannot also be a physical machine that is identical with every other human being. And if you are indeed unique, no physician can hold a master key to your health. Ayurveda recognizes this. That is why, when a vaidya says, "You're one in a billion," it is not meant to be a compliment; it is as simple a truth as saying that water is a fluid.

The logical question that arises from this is: if you are so totally unique, isn't pinpointing your unique maladies and their cures as difficult as trying to single out one particular wave in the Pacific Ocean? The ancient sages pondered the same question, and this led them to study the five elements more deeply.

Over time, the sages realized that the energies of the elements tend to work in pairs:

- According to Ayurvedic theory, fire needs moisture in order to burn, transform, and metabolize certain substances. When fire and moisture combine, as in corrosive liquids like acids or alkalis, they have the strength to transform, burn, and convert substances — that is why fiery pitta governs metabolism.
- Air needs ether, or space, in which to move.
- Earth is cemented by water, and water flows on a bed of earth.

They further observed that these energy pairs combine inside human beings:

- Ether and air combine to form the energy of propulsion or motion, which is called *vata* in Ayurveda.

- Fire and water combine to form the energy of metabolism, which is *pitta.*
- Earth and water combine to form the energy of solidity and structure, or *kapha.*

The sages next concluded that no two people shared exactly the same combination of these three energies; just as people had unique voices and faces, they also had unique energy patterns. Understanding these unique patterns, then, was the key to unlocking an individual's specific health problems.

So how did they classify these energy types? They called these three energies — vata, pitta, and kapha — the three doshas. The word *dosha* means "fault." So, in Ayurvedic terms, when any one or all of these three doshas are either impaired or aggravated, you have a dosha imbalance. In other words, there is a "fault" or "error" that needs correcting.

To find out which doshas in an individual needed correction, the sages had to first know what the individual's natural dosha combination was. This they did by assigning "dosha types" to people. Simply put, a person with more vata energy was called a "vata dosha type," while someone with more pitta attributes was a "pitta dosha type" of person, and so on.

Today, you'll find that books on Ayurveda refer to this basic individual constitution by various names: "dosha type," "body type," "personality type." Whatever its name, the purpose is to indicate what your dominant body-mind energy is.

the elementary you

By now, it is clear that the journey toward Ayurvedic healing and wholeness begins with the knowledge of your unique dosha type. Although it is best to see a vaidya for this, you can guess your own basic dosha type. The way to do this is to think about which of the five elements seem to be strongest in your personality. Start by answering this question: are you more fire, air, earth, ether, or water? Give me an instinctive answer.

- If you said "fire," it's likely that you perceive yourself as a strong, bold, hot-tempered person.
- If you said "earth," you probably think of yourself as stable, practical, and calm.
- If your answer was "air," you're likely to see yourself as active, indecisive, and restless.

This is exactly how the ancient sages reasoned.

Now study the following lists, giving yourself one point for each quality you think applies to you. The dosha with the most points is your dominant dosha.

Vata

1. I am light and thin of build.
2. I think and act quickly.
3. My skin is dry and feels cool to the touch.
4. I cannot stand cold, dry weather.
5. My hunger and digestion are irregular.

6. I'm quick to grasp new information, but also quick to forget.
7. I tend to worry.
8. I have a tendency toward constipation.
9. I get light, interrupted sleep at night.
10. Warm, cooked foods and hot beverages comfort me.

Pitta

1. I am of moderate build.
2. My appetite and digestion are both strong.
3. My favorite foods are cold, and I love iced beverages.
4. I absolutely cannot skip meals; it gives me acidity.
5. My complexion is reddish, and I tend to have moles and freckles.
6. I cannot stand hot weather.
7. I sometimes wake up in the wee hours of the morning and find it hard to go back to sleep.
8. My memory is steady.
9. I can be irritable and quick-tempered.
10. I am sharp and hardworking, but I tend to be a perfectionist.

Kapha

1. I am solid and heavy of build.
2. I have great strength and endurance.
3. I am slow and methodical in everything I do.
4. My skin is oily and smooth.
5. I have a calm, steady personality.

6. Though I am slow to grasp new information, I don't easily forget.

7. It takes a lot for me to lose my temper or get excited. ✓

8. I am a heavy sleeper, and can sleep for hours at a time.

9. My digestion is slow, but then my appetite is also mild.

10. I have lush, thick, dark hair. ✓.

Does your final score show two dominant doshas rather than one? If so, don't worry; you belong to the vast majority of people who have two strong doshas in their personality, with the third one being less active. Very few people are pure vata, pitta, or kapha, and even rarer are those with a tridoshic personality — that is, when all three doshas are almost equally strong.

Let me give you a sample score. Let's say you had eight vata points, seven pitta points, and nine kapha points; your dominant doshas would obviously be kapha and vata, in that order. Therefore, a vaidya would call you a kapha-vata. Using this example, it should now be easy for you to tell which of these ten doshic types you are:

1. vata
2. pitta
3. kapha
4. vata-pitta
5. pitta-vata
6. vata-kapha
7. kapha-vata

8. pitta-kapha
9. kapha-pitta
10. vata-pitta-kapha

In each case, the dosha mentioned first is your dominant dosha. Thus, vata-pitta and pitta-vata might sound similar, but they are not; one has a higher air quotient and the other a higher fire quotient.

What if you discover that you are a rare tridoshic, or vata-pitta-kapha type? Vaidyas say this is both good and bad news. The good news is that you were born with all five elements nearly balanced in your personality. The bad news is that tridoshic people can find it more difficult to maintain balance. Also, imbalances are more difficult to pinpoint and treat in people with no clearly dominant dosha.

Remember: whatever your dominant dosha, each of us has all three doshas in us. Existence is not possible without any one dosha. It is just that, in most people, one dosha seems to be less active than the other two.

I know what you are asking at this point: how does knowing my dosha type really help? It helps tremendously. Let's say you have just discovered you are a pitta-vata type of person. This tells you that the heating qualities of fire are dominant in your personality, followed by the dry qualities of air. In order to maintain good health, your primary goal should be to make sure that your pitta does not get aggravated. That is, you should eat cooling foods, avoid hot weather, and stay in the company of relaxed people who offset your intense personality. In addition, you should drink plenty of water, which not only cools pitta but also counters the dryness of vata dosha. This is, of course, just one example. Each dosha combination requires a different balancing strategy.

dosha imbalances

What happens when there is an imbalance? How will you know which of your doshas is out of balance? What can you do to correct it? For answers to these and similar questions, read the lists below:

Vata
When Vata Is In Balance:

- You are creative and full of enthusiasm;
- You make lots of friends, feel happy, and spread cheer;
- Your mind is clear and alert;
- Your bowels work well, and your urinary tract is healthy;
- Your bodily tissues function as they should;
- You sleep soundly and wake up refreshed;
- Your resistance to disease is good, and you feel energetic.

When Vata Is Out of Balance:

- You worry and fret;
- You're restless and easily tired;

- You tend to be oversensitive and indecisive;
- You cannot sleep;
- Your skin feels rough and dry;
- You start to lose weight and look gaunt;
- You suffer from constipation.

Typical Vata Complaints:

- Pain
- Cramps
- Chills
- Spasms

Your Vata Goes Out of Balance When:

- You exercise too much;
- You don't maintain a regular sleep pattern;
- You suffer a fall or fracture;
- You suppress natural urges, such as hunger, thirst, sleep, and sex;
- You are exposed to cold weather;
- You are grieving or afraid;
- You are angry or agitated;
- You observe a fast;
- You eat pungent, astringent, and bitter foods.

Vata Calmers:

- Get more warm, oily, heavy, sweet, sour, and salty foods in your diet;
- Reduce your intake of light, dry, cold, pungent, bitter, and astringent foods;
- Avoid stimulants like coffee and alcohol;

- Eat warm cooked foods;
- Be in warm environments;
- Give yourself a daily massage with a good-quality sesame oil;
- Go to bed early and follow a regular routine.

Pitta
When Pitta Is In Balance:

- You are focused and energetic;
- You are courageous and chivalrous;
- You are creative, organized, and often an excellent public speaker;
- Your heat and thirst mechanisms function well;
- Your complexion is lustrous;
- Your digestion is perfect;
- Your skin and body feel soft.

When Pitta Is Out of Balance:

- You tend to be sarcastic, impatient, and irritable;
- You can be bossy and tend to be a perfectionist;
- You don't get adequate sleep;
- Your complexion is yellowish;
- Your digestion is upset;
- Your body feels excessively hot;
- You suffer from inflammatory skin conditions.

Typical Pitta Complaints:

- Heartburn
- Soreness
- Fever

- Hot flashes
- Ulcers

Your Pitta Goes Out of Balance When:

- You are angry;
- The sun is too strong;
- You are fasting;
- You eat or use sesame or linseed products;
- Your diet is rich in sour foods, such as yogurt, wine, and vinegar;
- You're working too hard and straining to meet deadlines.

Pitta Pleasers:

- Use cooling spices such as fennel, coriander, and cardamom in your cooking;
- Take cool baths;
- Avoid hot temperatures and hot food;
- Drink plenty of water;
- Find time to relax and do things you like;
- Don't overwork;
- Eat your meals — especially lunch — on time.

Kapha
When Kapha Is In Balance:

- You feel stable in mind;
- You act with courage and dignity;
- You feel affectionate and forgiving toward others;
- You feel strong;
- You are filled with energy;

- Your joints are well lubricated and supple;
- Your body is well proportioned.

When Kapha Is Out of Balance:

- You feel lethargic and lack motivation;
- You tend to oversleep;
- Your joints feel loose;
- You gain excessive weight;
- You suffer from respiratory problems;
- Your sinuses trouble you;
- Your complexion is pale;
- You feel cold.

Typical Kapha Complaints:

- Congestion
- Fluid retention
- Lethargy
- Joint pain

Your Kapha Goes Out of Balance When:

- You sleep during the day;
- You are depressed;
- You eat heavy, rich food;
- Your diet is heavy in sweet, sour, or salty foods;
- You consume a lot of dairy products.

Kapha Controllers:

- Follow a kapha-regulating diet prescribed by a vaidya;

- Apply wet-heat fomentation, such as a warm sesame oil massage;
- Get more exercise;
- Get fewer hours of sleep, with no daytime naps.

the four dos of dosha-watching

1. Do consult a vaidya. Although charts and questionnaires make the job of identifying your dosha type quick and easy, it is always best to have your pulse read by a qualified Ayurvedic physician whose trained eye will give you the most accurate assessment of your dosha type and who will suggest ways to balance those that are depleted or in excess.

2. Do try to deduce your own doshas, too. Though I just said that a vaidya is best qualified to assess your doshas, there's every reason you should also take a self-assessment quiz from time to time. This helps you get in touch with your changing preferences, emotions, and habits — which, in turn, affect the balance of your doshas. Further, answering such questions can point your attention to small problems you might have been ignoring.

3. Do observe people around you and try to figure out their dosha types. This will help you develop a better understanding of how the doshas work and make them seem more real to you. Look

around; your plump, placid, matronly neighbor who is always baking you cookies is likely to be a kapha type. Your boss, with the perpetually protruding vein on her forehead, is probably a pitta personality. Your stick-thin friend who flits from topic to topic within minutes and can never seem to decide on anything is Madame vata.

Learning about people and their doshas yields a nice little benefit: it can help you understand why people behave the way they do. And to understand, said a wise man, is to forgive. Therefore, the next time you feel exasperated with your indecisive friend, you can say to yourself, "It's not her, it's her vata in action!" Then, with the help of chapter 13, "Living Ayurveda, Giving Ayurveda," you can think up ways to appease your friend's restless dosha.

4. Do remember that the doshas are complex. The lists and questions are really surface guides to help you understand the ABCs of the doshas.

In the next chapter, we will study the doshas and their behavior more closely. Only after reading that material should you start delving more deeply into your own doshic personality.

learning the language of the elements

If the doors of perception were cleansed,
everything would appear to man as it is: infinite.

— William Blake

Watch water boiling in a pot. What makes it start boiling at a particular moment? On the face of it, it is the intensity of the flame underneath. But think a little more deeply, and you will come up with many other factors: the altitude at which the kitchen is located, the width of the pot, whether or not the pot is covered with a lid, the initial temperature of the water, and so on.

Similarly, scores of factors determine how your doshas behave at any given point. That is why it is unwise to try to analyze your doshas using simplistic charts; they're too complex for that.

Consider the diverse forces that play upon your doshas moment by moment:

- the events of your day
- the recent events in your life
- your current lifestyle: diet, sleep patterns, work routine
- the time of day
- the season of the year
- your age

The result: you cannot look on a chart and immediately say, "My sleep is disturbed so I need to reduce my vata dosha." The thing to do is to find out which factors have come together to disturb your sleep. Is it that you have been napping in the afternoons? Are you bogged down by work? Has there been a conflict in your family life? Is your room heater set to an uncomfortable temperature? Or is it that you've just turned sixty, when sleep is known to become erratic? Is it just vata, or is it a combination of doshas at fault here?

Admittedly, discovering this multitude of dosha-manipulating factors can leave you somewhat bemused, like the centipede in this rhyme:

The centipede was happy, quite
until a frog in fun
said, "Pray, which leg comes after which?"
which raised her mind to such a pitch

she lay distracted in a ditch
considering how to run.

Don't worry! Your dilemma is going to be nowhere as vexing as that of the centipede. The factors that affect your doshas are quite easy to understand because, like everything else in Ayurveda, the doshas are based on common sense and practical logic. In fact, after reading this chapter, you will have a good idea of what makes the quality and impact of your doshas fluctuate.

dosha climate, dosha weather

Let me begin with a somewhat surprising statement: Your dosha type is really two dosha types, one you are born with and another that changes constantly. Your original dosha makeup was decided the moment you were conceived. You were born with it, and it will remain constant throughout your life. In Sanskrit, your basic dosha type is called your *prakriti*, or nature.

However, season, time, and circumstance constantly act upon and change this original combination of energies, and this ever-in-flux dosha makeup is what vaidyas call *vikriti*, or distortion.

The difference between prakriti and vikriti is exactly like that between climate and weather. The "climate," or prakriti, of your being consists of the constant factors: your bone structure, food preferences, and emotional makeup, to name a few.

But the vikriti, or "weather," of your personality changes all the time, affecting such daily rhythms as appetite, moods, and energy levels. Although the meaning of vikriti — distortion — might lead you to believe otherwise, life would be all wrong without vikriti; imagine feeling equally hungry, happy, lethargic, or enthusiastic all the time!

In real life, your prakriti and vikriti both affect what you do and how you feel at any given time. For example, if you were born with a strong vata dosha, you tend to feel the cold more than others. This affects the choices you make in daily life. On a cold day, you'll want to stay indoors and treat yourself to warm soup while your pitta friend is out skiing.

Different dosha types seek different ways to balance themselves. A tired pitta finds relief in a cool shower. Vata people benefit greatly from a moisturizing massage. An easy-paced walk can restore sagging kapha spirits. Thus, whatever your preferred idea of relaxation, you are essentially seeking to come closer to your original dosha makeup, or prakriti. This is a very happy state to be in, for Ayurvedic healers know that living in harmony with your innate qualities is the key to living a happy, healthy life.

This dosha-friendly approach to living helps in a much broader sense, too. For example, a person whose basic dosha type is kapha would enjoy and excel at a relatively low-stress job, while vata would love a creative environment and pitta would thrive in a dynamic one.

Obviously, then, setting out to "balance your doshas" does not mean striving for equal amounts of vata, pitta, and kapha in your life; that can almost never be. Life is so fluid that dosha balancing just means trying to get your vikriti as close as possible to your original dosha type, or prakriti. Once you understand the doshas more fully, this will be easy to achieve.

the doshas around you

Would you ever imagine 2:00 A.M. as being governed by a dosha? How about February being a certain dosha type? The ancient sages who wrote Ayurvedic texts imagined just that. Because they saw humans and the cosmos as an integrated whole, they ascribed the same dosha attributes to nature and its cycles.

The Doshas in a Twenty-Four-Hour Day

Early in the morning, the sky is bewitchingly beautiful and all of nature is beginning to fill up with fresh energy. By afternoon, energy levels peak and appetite is sharp. In the evening we head home from work, while the birds fly back to their nests. Then comes the night, with its balm of restful sleep. These natural rhythms echo the qualities of the three doshas — one restless, another intense, and the third calm. In accordance with these rhythms, Ayurvedic philosophy divides the twenty-four-hour day into distinct dosha zones:

- **Vata Time:** 2:00 to 6:00 A.M. and 2:00 to 6:00 P.M. The early hours of the morning and evening are ideal for active and creative work.

That is why Ayurvedic practitioners recommend rising in "vata time." If you sleep late, you will feel dull and groggy because you have stepped into the next zone, which is "kapha time."

- **Kapha Time:** 6:00 to 10:00 A.M. and 6:00 to 10:00 P.M. Both of these are periods when your activity levels are either slowly increasing or slowly winding down. Therefore, rising after 6:00 A.M. or not going to bed between 6:00 and 10:00 P.M. can cause disturbed sleep.

- **Pitta Time:** 10:00 A.M. to 2:00 P.M. and 10:00 P.M. to 2:00 A.M. Fiery pitta governs the productive hours from midmorning to the middle of the day, and again late in the night when the digestive system is busy processing and assimilating dinner.

One way you can use this information is to tell whether your dosha imbalance is related to the time of day. For example, if you find it difficult to stay awake in the mornings without three cups of coffee, it could be because you have been rising late — during the lethargic kapha time. Try waking up an hour earlier, and your mornings will be filled with verve.

The Doshas in a Twelve-Month Year

Just as the doshas shift duties during a single day, they also govern the rhythm of the seasons. Here's the Seasonal Dosha Chart:

Vata season: mid-October to mid-February
Kapha season: mid-February to mid-June
Pitta season: mid-June to mid-October

Here are some tips that will help you through the seasons. They will also balance your doshas in general. That is, the tips for cooling pitta in summer are beneficial to pitta year-round, and similarly for vata and kapha.

How to Soothe Pitta in Summer

The humid, intense heat of summer makes it pitta season. At this time of the year, the heat can make us more prone to irritability and temper outbursts. This is when pitta-related skin and digestion problems (acne, heat rashes, acidity, heartburn) flare up, too. Even kapha-vata types can suffer from heat rashes, dry skin, and excessive thirst in summer. Once you understand this summer-pitta link, it becomes both important and easy to find ways to beat the heat.

1. Eat as many sweet, ripe, juicy fruits as you can between July and October: apples, pears, melons, and mangoes. Their cooling nectar keeps the body hydrated and happy.

2. Get more vegetables such as broccoli, cucumber, zucchini, and carrots in your diet; they are considered to have cooling properties, too.

3. Use spices such as mint, fennel, and coriander, which also have cooling properties. In the summer season, they're your best friends. Mustard seeds and ginger, on the other hand, have a

heating effect on the metabolism — which is not desirable at this time.

4. Try to avoid such foods as yogurt, cayenne pepper, and sour cream while summer lasts. A heat-distraught pitta does not enjoy sour, salty, and very spicy foods — especially at this time of the year.

5. Resist the urge to ice your drinks. Though, in general, liquid, lukewarm, or cool foods are more comforting in summer than hot, dry ones, the frigidity of ice douses digestive fire.

6. Take a swim, go ice skating, or stroll in the moonlight. Pick cooling exercises like these to keep pitta from flaring up.

Wise Ways to Balance Vata in Winter

In winter, the air is dry and cool — both qualities of vata. Though many of us dread the winter months for the fat they pile up around our waists, Ayurvedic healers see winter as an excellent time to nourish the body and build immunity through wholesome food and a healthy routine.

1. Eat foods that please the vata dosha: sweet, warm, lubricating foods cooked in easy-to-digest oils such as olive oil or ghee (clarified butter).

2. Cook with spices like cumin, ginger, and turmeric at this time. They support digestion and boost immunity.

3. Combat the dryness of these vata months by regularly massaging and moisturizing your skin and drinking warm water (if you are a pitta type, room-temperature water is fine).

4. Include plenty of fresh fruits and vegetables in your diet.

5. Take a warm bath or shower every winter morning; this is especially energizing because it opens the pores, removing toxins. Preceded by an herbalized oil massage, its benefits increase manifold.

Healing Things to Do in Spring

In spring, ice thaws, blossoms unfold, and spirits soar. At the same time, accumulated toxins of winter start to liquefy naturally, too. With a little help from you, this flushing out of impurities can be even more efficient.

1. Eat light, nongreasy foods that detoxify the body, thus appeasing the kapha dosha that rules this season.

2. Include increased servings of whole grains and cooked leafy greens in your diet.

3. Maintain a good skin routine: cleanse, tone, and moisturize morning and evening, and exfoliate twice a week to remove dead cells and open pores. (See chapter 10 for specific recommendations.)

4. Regulate your bowel habits. If you have been irregular, now is the time to pay special attention to this aspect of your day. Remember,

spring is detox season. Drink warm water before you attempt a bowel movement. Don't worry if regularity does not return within a day or even a week. Give it time, but don't give up.

The Seasons of Your Life

The three doshas are also programmed to govern the different phases of your life in turns.

- Kapha rules infancy and childhood — the formative years.
- Pitta governs adulthood through middle age — the productive years.
- Vata increases with old age — the years when sleep becomes lighter and erratic, the skin loses moisture, and the joints stiffen.

the doshas and their deputies

What makes the doshas slightly more complex is that each of them has five deputies called *subdoshas*. Each subdosha, according to Ayurvedic practice, has a specific location and a specific set of duties. (You can think of them as state governments.) At first glance, the sheer number of the subdoshas and their unfamiliar names can seem confusing, but to a vaidya the subdoshas are invaluable. When a dosha misbehaves, the vaidya can go deeper and tell exactly which aspect of that dosha is disturbed and how it can be brought back on track.

Here is a list of the subdoshas and their jurisdictions.

You do not need to memorize them; I'm enumerating them just to show you that they are less complex than they first seem, but at the same time vital to Ayurvedic healing:

Vata Subdoshas
Prana Vata

Prana means "life force." That is why you could call the prana vata the chief subdosha among all fifteen. Located in the head, heart, chest, and sense organs, prana vata governs vision, hearing, smell, taste, creative thinking, reasoning, and enthusiasm.

Udana Vata

Udana means "upward moving." Hence, udana vata is responsible for quality of voice, memory, and movement of thought. A speech defect would indicate a weakened udana vata.

Samana Vata

Samana means "balancing" or "equalizing." This subdosha resides in the middle region of the body, including the navel, stomach, and small intestine. Therefore, its function is to fan the fires of digestion or assist the agni of pitta in the digestive process.

Apana Vata

Apana means "downward moving." The apana vata sits in the nether regions and regulates the flow of waste, ejaculate, and menstrual fluid.

Vyana Vata

Vyana (vi-ana) means the "diffusive" or "pervasive." *Vi* is a prefix meaning "apart" or "to separate." Though this subdosha is indeed present all over the body, its primary seat is the heart. Blood flow, heart rhythm, perspiration, the sense of touch — all these are vyana vata responsibilities.

Pitta Subdoshas
Alochaka Pitta

Alochaka means "critic" — the fire that can "criticize," or in another sense, "perceive" visually. This subdosha is located in the eyes and governs vision. In youth, the alochaka pitta is generally strong. Toward old age, it becomes weakened, causing all sorts of problems ranging from eye strain to cataracts.

Bhrajaka Pitta

A close meaning of the word *bhrajaka* is "to diffuse" — or "spread." This is the subdosha that lends radiance to your skin. On the other hand, a disturbed bhrajaka pitta could lead to allergies, rashes, and skin inflammation.

Sadhaka Pitta

Sadhaka means the fire that helps us recognize the truth or reality, from the root *sadh*, meaning "to accomplish" or "to realize." Fortunate is the person whose sadhaka pitta is balanced, for this heart-based subdosha metabolizes thought and feeling. Thus, key areas of your life, such as desire, drive, decisiveness, and spirituality, are under the care of the sadhaka pitta.

Pachaka Pitta

Pachaka comes from the root word *pachan*, or "digestion." How well you digest, assimilate, and metabolize
the food you eat depends on how balanced your pachaka
pitta is.

Ranjaka Pitta

Ranjaka means "that which colors." Your biggest
organ — the liver — is governed by this subdosha. So
are the spleen and stomach. Therefore, the rich red color
of your blood and its healthy and toxin-free flow are
functions of ranjaka pitta.

Kapha Subdoshas
Tarpaka Kapha

The word *tarpaka* is derived from *tripti,* which
means "contentment." Thus, tarpaka kapha means the
form of water that gives contentment. This subdosha
nourishes the nose, mouth, eyes, and brain. It is
responsible for good lubrication of the nostrils, eyes,
and cerebrospinal column. As an extension of these
responsibilities, tarpaka kapha also influences emotional well-being.

Bodhaka Kapha

Bodh means "awareness," therefore bodhaka kapha
means the form of water that helps us perceive taste — the
first stage of digestion. Bodhaka kapha is the subdosha that
helps us discriminate the strong and subtle flavors that our
taste buds encounter. A "metallic" taste in the mouth is a
typical symptom of a weakened bodhaka kapha.

Kledaka Kapha

Kledaka kapha means the form of water that moistens. Lubrication is an important part of the digestive process. Without the enzymes and juices that go to work on food, there would be no digestion at all. Kledaka kapha makes sure these juices are in rich supply.

Avalambaka Kapha

Avalamb means "support." Therefore, avalambaka kapha means the form of water that gives support. Indeed, all other subdoshas depend on the support of avalambaka kapha for moisture. The very plasma inside a cell is made of this subdosha, which also protects the heart, strengthens the muscles, and looks after the health of the lungs.

Sleshaka Kapha

Sleshaka comes from the root word *slish*, which means to be moist or sticky. Stiff, creaky joints are often the result of a disturbed sleshaka kapha. This subdosha is located in the joints as the synovial fluid and is responsible for holding them together and promoting ease of movement.

who's the moodiest of them all?

Again, the above list of subdoshas was just to introduce you to them. When you are new to Ayurveda, you need only concern yourself chiefly with the three parent doshas:

- Vata, which governs movement
- Pitta, which rules metabolism, and
- Kapha, which looks after structure and frame

If there were an "ideal quantity guide to the doshas" — that is, something like thirty units each of vata, pitta, and kapha for perfect health — we would have by now found a way to tell exactly how many units short or in excess we were. But not only are the doshas not quantifiable, they are also invisible. Therefore, trying to tell which one of them is acting up can be tricky.

However, there are clues. One major generalization vaidyas have been able to make is that most disease stems from a disorder in one particular dosha. Can you guess which one it is?

The logical answer, of course, is vata, which combines the restless and volatile energies of air and ether. Therefore, people whose vata dosha is dominant from birth are prone to suffer many more health problems than the other two dosha types. Restlessness, anxiety, poor digestion, fatigue, aches, and pains — a disturbed vata can produce a plethora of symptoms.

On the other hand, this knowledge poses the danger of misdiagnosis. Let's say you have stiff joints. While excess vata can indeed cause joint stiffness, it is kapha that is responsible for joint lubrication — and your condition could mean that your kapha dosha is weak. Now, if you jumped to the conclusion that your problem is vata related, some of your vata-balancing measures could actually worsen the kapha disorder, making those joints even stiffer.

There's more. Often, two doshas will go out of control at the same time or close upon each other's heels. If you are unable to sleep because you are deeply angry with someone, both your vata and your pitta are not in equilibrium. And a disease like asthma takes root when all three doshas are out of balance.

the mind and the doshas

In Western medicine, you are as healthy as your last clinical exam. That is, as long as your cholesterol levels and blood pressure are normal, your X ray is clear, and your heartbeat is regular, you are considered to be in good health. The standard checkup does not measure or assess the quality of your mental and emotional health. That is why the exam is called a "physical" — and, of course, there is no such thing as an annual "mental."

But because Ayurveda is equally concerned with the health of body and mind, its healers have studied the dosha-mind connection in great detail.

Take depression. First of all, the triggers of depression in all three dosha types are very different. Secondly, each dosha type experiences depression differently. Vatas tend to get depressed as a result of excess strain, fear, shock, grief, or addiction. Pittas are likely to suffer depression when they drive themselves too hard, harbor resentment or anger toward someone, expect too much from others and fail to get it, or become fussy perfectionists. Kaphas, who are normally calm and unruffled, can go into deep depression if their relationships are not fulfilling enough. Kapha is by nature possessive, and can become clingy and dependent if unbalanced. Also, kapha cannot easily accept change, so major changes in people and things make a kapha type of person feel forlorn and pessimistic.

As you can see, taming the doshas by trying to tabulate their whims is not a great idea. They are too complex for that. But at the same time, the whole idea in Ayurveda is to help oneself. So what does one do?

Plenty! There are three things you can do — and understand — at this point:

1. Go to a vaidya who, through training in pulse diagnosis, will make an accurate assessment of your dosha type and your imbalances. Keeping all the varied factors in mind — your personality, the environment, the seasons — the vaidya will give you the gist of his findings. This will not only point out the specific areas that need attention, but will also give you practical solutions to get your systems back into harmony.

2. Call upon your invaluable intuitive powers to guide you toward balance. It's easy; nature is helping you do it anyway. When it is cold, you switch on the heater. If it is summer, you feel more thirsty and drink more liquids. All you have to do is obey nature more often. If you are hungry, put work on hold and eat. If you are stressed, don't get angry — get refreshed.

3. There is such a thing as a single recipe for perfect balance without worrying about the intricacies. What's more, it is something you will love doing. Whatever the circumstances or season, you can please all your doshas by doing just one simple thing: follow a nature-friendly routine.

What is a "nature-friendly" routine? It's a routine that imitates both nature's daily rhythm and its seasonal rhythm: day-night, spring-summer-fall-winter, birth-and-death. The ancient sages who studied Ayurveda saw in that rhythm something more than a pattern; they found in it the key to human happiness.

We shall unlock the best of those happy secrets in the next chapter.

routine matters – and how!

And if tonight my soul may find her peace in sleep, and sink in good oblivion, and in the morning wake like a new-opened flower then I have been dipped again in God, and new-created.

— D. H. Lawrence

If I had to choose the most important chapter in this book, I would pick this one without hesitation. The reason is: if you read no other chapter but this one, you will have learned how to "do" Ayurveda. Regardless of your dosha type, prakriti or vikriti, you can follow the advice here to achieve that elusive thing — balance — in your life with the utmost ease.

Let me start by telling you about a man I used to know — a man who lived a life very close to the Ayurvedic ideal.

an ordinary man

As children, we often spent the summer vacation with our grandparents, who lived in a lovely little earth-scented village. Every night, I would resolve to watch the dawn, which Grandpa told me was breathtaking against the cornstalks. I am ashamed to say that I always woke up long after the roosters had finished crowing. By that time, the sun would be high in the sky, and Grandpa hard at work in the fields.

It is about Grandpa that I want to tell you.

My grandfather never popped a pill. At the ripe young age of eighty-seven, he rose daily under a still-inky sky. Be it January or July, he bathed under a gushing tap of ice-cold water in the verandah, wearing only a muslin loincloth. He chewed on a twig from a neem tree to clean his teeth and strengthen his gums. After his ablutions, he would do yoga exercises. Village folk looked up to him — quite literally, for he was tall and strong, with a booming voice.

Grandma complemented her husband's energy perfectly. By the time he was ready for breakfast, at about 7:00 A.M., she would be bathed and ready, too — with a hearty meal of fresh griddle bread and hot vegetable curry, laden with dollops of homemade ghee.

No one was surprised when, one night, Grandpa and Grandma fought off and captured three robbers who broke into their farmhouse. Vaidyas would give the credit to my grandparents' *dincharya* (*din:* "day," *charya:*

"to follow"), or daily routine, which moved in perfect rhythm with nature's own clock.

nature's unseen clock

How punctually the sun tiptoes up, then shines boldly overhead, and finally climbs down the sky. How unfailingly the birds twitter out of their nests, gather food all day, and slip back home as dusk falls. Of course these eternal rhythms are wondrous in themselves, but they can take on new meaning if you stop to think about them in the context of your own life.

Think about it. Given a choice, your body would follow a similar rhythm. Your lungs would love to fill up with the fresh morning air. Your stomach would welcome a complete meal at noon, when both appetite and digestive power are at their peak. After an early dinner, your mind and body would like to settle down for the night.

But, alas, we don't often allow ourselves such luxuries. When the sun sets, we surround ourselves with bright indoor lights. When the mind asks to rest, we force it to watch a late-night film. Lunch is often a cold, hurried affair — grabbed between meetings.

I happened to point this out to a friend who had been "grabbing" lunch for five years. She saw red. "Tell me something," she demanded, "what does Ayurveda expect you to do? Not attend meetings, not earn a living? This is not France, where everything shuts down at lunchtime!" I refrained from pointing out to her that their leisurely lunch could be a major reason why the French suffer fewer heart attacks — even though they eat four times more butter — than Americans do.

But then I do understand what she means. Right now, when life is a daily struggle to take in a full breath — let alone a fresh meal — it does seem a little unreasonable to work at changing a whole lifestyle. But then that is why I admire Ayurveda so much; it never asks you to wipe your slate clean and begin afresh. Being the user-friendly system of healing that it is, Ayurveda asks you to introduce change slowly and comfortably until your healthy new habits weave themselves into your daily routine.

There are two good reasons why the vaidya does not want you to rush into lifestyle changes. First, forced change is like a crash diet or a sudden storm; it won't last. Second, compelling yourself to adjust to a new routine, even if it's beneficial to you, is in itself a source of stress to the mind — and stress of any kind is against Ayurvedic principles.

Therefore, Ayurveda invites you to discover your healthier self, step by baby step.

the recharging routine

Delicious! That's the word I would use to describe the ideal Ayurvedic routine, which is built not to suit other people — clients, boss, friends, spouse, child — but to please the one person who matters most in your life: YOU. This, to me, is its unique selling point.

Going back to Grandfather's daily routine, let us admit that he was able to follow it because he lived so close to nature. Had he been a big-city executive, his appointment book might have looked something like this:

9:00 Board meeting
11:00 Briefing/teleconference
1:00 Luncheon meeting
2:00 Discussions with delegates
5:00 Addressing press conference
7:00 Rotary Club speech

An admirer of success is sure to see in this diary an enviable lifestyle. A vaidya would see in it an arduous one, guaranteed to produce tons of disorder-causing ama. Everything in this person's day obviously revolves around other people, and that is not just because he or she is such a busy executive. Whatever your profession or situation, your lifestyle is probably not tailor-made for you.

When I was a television journalist in India, for instance, I did not even have a fixed schedule. I would have given anything to have one! News of a raging fire or a sudden political crisis meant that I went without a bath, breakfast, lunch — sometimes dinner, too.

Even today, when I have a more relaxed job, my weekends are seldom my own. They start with making breakfast for the family and end with making lunch for Monday. In between, I clean the bathrooms, make beds, and shop for groceries. Any time that I want purely for myself, I have to steal. I am sure I am echoing a story everyone has heard.

The question I am asking here is, What space or time do you and I keep in our day for an appointment with ourselves? As far as Ayurveda is concerned, this is a question of supreme importance, and the answer should ideally be: All day! This is, of course, not to say that we should shrink into ourselves and forget about everyone and everything else. The logic of the vaidya is: only when you are centered in yourself can you establish a truly meaningful relationship with the world.

Think about it, and the meaning of this plain statement will shine clearly before you. When you wake up groggy and rush out of the house without breakfast, you cannot expect to give your best to the meeting in progress. With your nerves stretched like ropes inside your head, you cannot hope to spread cheer among friends and family.

The solution, as I said, is delicious.

reinvent your day

How about acting as your own personal secretary and rescheduling your appointment book not by your wrist-watch but by nature's clock?

That is, what if your daily planner looked like this?

Arise with the Sun

The light-and-swift vata dosha dominates the early morning hours, making it an ideal time for you to start your day. Arise early, ideally by 6:00 or before the sun rises. At this glorious hour, all of nature is waking up —

the sun, the birds, the flowers. The air is fresh and calm. Your body and mind are rested and ready for renewal. Your organs of elimination are ready to shed yesterday's waste. There is in this hour a purity, a godliness in nature that your spirit will love.

Before you leave your bed, take a few moments to think sunny thoughts about the day that stretches ahead. I am reminded here of the words of English writer Monica Baldwin: "The moment when you first wake up in the morning, you possess the certainty that, during the day that lies before you, absolutely anything may happen. And the fact that it practically always doesn't, matters not a jot. The possibility is always there."

If you have a baby who keeps you awake through the night, or young kids who demand all of your attention in the morning, you could try to get your kids in bed early. That way, you might soon develop a rhythm of waking up half an hour before they do. It will give you peace and quiet for thirty minutes, as well as a head start on your day.

If you work night shifts, however, you might want to sleep through the morning — and that would be perfectly justified. Also, vaidyas recommend drinking plenty of water if you have been working in the late-night pitta hours; this keeps digestion smooth.

Whatever you do, don't push yourself into an early-rising routine; that will only be an additional strain, and the point of Ayurveda is not to strain you in any way.

Freshen Up

Pay attention to those small ablutions; they are big on health benefits. Wash your face. Clean your eyes, nose, and mouth. Stick out your tongue and look at it in the mirror. Is it coated with white? That's a visible sign of ama, or undigested toxic matter. If it stays there, your breath will feel stale and your taste buds will be unable to do their job. Scrape your tongue with a specially designed silver or stainless steel scraper, called a tongue cleaner or tongue scraper (see resources for buying information), working back to front six or seven times. Feel your breath freshen instantly. According to vaidyas, this scraping action also ignites the body's engine, so to speak, preparing it to perform its daily job of respiration, circulation, digestion, and elimination more efficiently.

Irrigate Your Body

Drink a full of glass of warm water. This will get your kidneys and bowels ready for evacuation. If a rushed routine has you accustomed to an irregular bowel movement, don't try to get it back to regularity in a hurry. Reestablishing the morning rhythm will take time. Five minutes after you drink warm water, try to have a bowel movement. If it does not happen, don't worry; within the next few days, you will probably be able to regularize this vital part of your healthy routine.

Rub Your Body Awake

Early morning being vata time, your skin tends to be dry. Give it moisture and suppleness by massaging in a good-quality Ayurvedic oil; cold-pressed, chemical-free, organic sesame oil works best. If you are new to self-massage, you only have to try it once to understand its benefits. I know of no other therapy that can so quickly both fill you with energy and make you feel totally rested. Massage accomplishes this by boosting your circulation while simultaneously calming your nervous system.

Ayurvedic healers have prepared a step-by-step massage technique, designed to give you the maximum benefit from this morning routine. You will find this complete technique in chapter 10.

Make Time to Take a Walk

Long before exercise became a modern mantra, Ayurveda's founding father, Sage Charaka, was singing generous praises of it. He lauded its capacity to burn ama, restore "flow" to the body's essential channels, strengthen the mind, and even delay aging. Daily exercise has, therefore, always been a vital part of the ideal Ayurvedic routine.

But, vaidyas caution, there is such a thing as too much exercise. People who fight too hard to be fit defy one of the most basic Ayurvedic rules: moderation in everything. The result? Instead of feeling energized, they feel exhausted. And by stretching their muscles too far, they disturb their overall balance instead of restoring it.

So let your rule of thumb be to spend only half of your available energy reserve at one time. There is no calculator or monitor that can tell you when you've used up 50 percent of your reserve, but your body will give you signals. If you can keep up conversation while walking, feel light and lively after your workout, and enjoy your game of tennis, your body is happy. But if you're sweating profusely, breathing through your mouth, and starting to feel exhausted, it is time to stop. It's really that simple.

Before breakfast is the ideal time to get your morning exercise. Some forms of exercise, such as a brisk twenty-minute walk and simple yoga asanas, balance all three doshas and are considered ideal.

Be Good to Yourself — Eat Breakfast

"Never leave home on an empty stomach." Grandmothers in India have said this for so many generations that it has taken on the status of folklore. When you read about Ayurveda, you come to understand the reason for the Indian grandmothers' insistence on breakfast.

After it has been awakened and cleansed, the human body needs to be nourished. If you deprive it of that nutrition, it will produce acid and make you feel uncomfortable. Come noon, the digestive fire will rise, adding to the acid levels and making you feel uncomfortable. In addition, missing out on breakfast disturbs sadhaka pitta, the subdosha that looks after emotions — particularly the feelings of comfort and contentment. If you miss breakfast regularly, you will eventually disturb the balance of all three doshas.

But the good news is that you can restore that lost balance quite easily if you work your way back to a good morning meal. As with everything else, go slowly in breaking the no-breakfast habit. Start with a fresh fruit or vegetable juice and gradually get your stomach accustomed to such foods as almonds or raisins soaked overnight in water, warm bread with honey, cooked cereal, and fresh juicy fruit of your choice.

Most of us don't think twice about following up a bowl of cereal or a cup of coffee with a glass of juice. The Ayurvedic practice, however, is to not combine milk with acidic foods such as sour fruit, yogurt, or cheese. The acidic properties of these foods, it is believed, curdle the milk in the stomach. This can result in disturbed digestion. Moreover — and this might come as a surprise — drinking orange juice first thing in the morning is a kind of acid assault on the stomach; it is better to drink it later in the day. A nourishing alternative is to start your day with a stewed apple or pear. In chapter 9, I will describe the method of preparing stewed fruit.

About coffee: vaidyas advise avoiding caffeinated beverages altogether, but if you find that impossible to do, then at least limit your intake to two cups a day. If you take milk in your coffee, boil it first; doing this is believed to reduce the side effects of caffeine to some extent.

Wash your hands before and after eating. Clean your teeth and tongue after every meal. If possible, get some gentle exercise after eating, such as a brief stroll, to aid digestion. Apply a soothing Ayurvedic perfume, made from essential oils. Dress with care; the color and texture of your clothes should reflect the harmony within you. These things may sound obvious — even trivial — but it is surprising how many of us neglect to do them the way they should be done.

Eat Lunch Like a King

Lunch deserves to be your largest meal of the day because afternoon is when two powerful forces are at their peak: the energy of the sun, and the "fire" of your digestion. Even if you work in an office, you needn't be stuck with choosing between a sandwich and, well, a sandwich. With a little planning, you can treat yourself to a hot, fresh meal at work by using a slow-cooker. Just put fresh vegetables and the grains of your choice into the cooker in the morning, and by lunchtime you will have a healthful soup ready.

Here are some general guidelines on lunch: Ayurvedic philosophy says that the ideal quantity of food for a single meal is the amount that can be scooped up with both hands. Don't gobble; chew. Be aware of the food you are eating; concentrate on it. If possible, eat in silence without talking or laughing — and certainly without arguing. You'll help your metabolic process.

The often-asked question is: to drink or not to drink water with your meal? Vaidyas say it is okay to sip a cup of room-temperature or warm water during your meal. If your meal is too dry, you can drink more than that. If you are drinking soup or lentils with lunch, then keep it to one cup. Drinking water about forty-five minutes after lunch is also good because it gives digestion a boost. Generally, drinking water at regular intervals through the day will work wonders for you.

Snacking between meals can lead to an erratic appetite, but as long as your last meal is fully digested before you snack, it won't harm you. When the urge to snack attacks, quickly think back to your last meal; if you ate it less than four hours ago, skip the snack.

Have an Early Dinner

Eating by about 7:00 P.M. is ideal, and allows time for your dinner to be properly digested before going to bed. Keep this meal light: soups, one-pot vegetable stews, quick-cooking grains like buckwheat, and sautéed vegetables make nourishing yet non-heavy dinners. Whenever possible, go for a gentle walk (around thirty minutes) before retiring.

Make Bedtime the Stuff of Dreams

Relax with light music, or lie in bed and breathe deeply, until you feel calm and mentally settled. Reading a book before bedtime can sometimes stimulate the mind instead of settling it, thus interfering with good sleep. Ideally, lights should be out at 10:00. The best sleeping position is on your side with knees slightly bent. Avoid sleeping on your stomach.

---

your ayurvedic day

There! You now have a pleasant, nurturing routine, as opposed to the "routine" routine you had been following. Isn't it surprising how much more you can squeeze into your day and still depressurize your life instead of cramming it with stress?

In between these essentials, you would, of course, fit

in your work-related appointments. Pepper the margins of your planner with interesting tips, reminders, and positive affirmations. A sampling:

- Refreshing Reminder: drink two extra glasses of water tomorrow.
- Note to Myself: Today I am a symphony of health and joy. I'm tuning the strings of my violin. I'm learning to realign my priorities and take life day by organized day. That is why the press conference figures second. My breakfast figures first.

Rewriting your appointment book in this way can help you live Ayurvedically every single day. And to live Ayurvedically is to live a long, happy, fulfilled life. Of course, there will be times when you cannot keep up with your Ayurvedic routine. Don't let that frustrate you. Accept the breaks just as you've learned to accept commercials interrupting your favorite television show. They're part of life. Be patient, and learn to calmly pick up the threads afresh.

Have a happy, healing, Ayurvedic day!

the delicious route
to healing

*My kitchen is a mystical place, a kind of temple for me.
It is a place where the surfaces seem to have significance,
where the sounds and odors carry meaning that transfers
from the past and bridges to the future.*

— Pearl Bailey

Before we talk about Ayurveda and its food philosophy, let us travel twenty years back and a few thou-
sand miles away to an apartment complex in New Delhi,
where the stars are still shining, the air is crisp, and the
streets are quiet. In this predawn hour, my mother rises
from bed.

Fifteen minutes later, she is kneading the dough to
make bread. Meanwhile, lightly spiced fresh green peas
sizzle in the wok. The school bus arrives in twenty minutes, but that is enough time for Mom's practiced hands

to cook and pack a complete meal for both my brother and me.

By the time the first ray of sunlight peeks into our living room, our mother has bathed and said her morning prayers. Soon a familiar sing-song voice floats across the street into her waiting ears:

"Lo aa gayi taazi subah ki mirchi, gobhi, palak." (Hindi for "Here's your morning supply of fresh peppers, cauliflower, and spinach leaves.")

Mom sprints down the stairs armed with an empty basket, a few rupee notes, and vocal cords ready for exercise (this last being essential for haggling with the vegetable vendor over the prices). Many energetic exchanges later, she waltzes back up, her basket brimming with vegetables and fruits in all shades of red, orange, yellow, and green.

Domestic help is readily available in India, but my mother prefers to do the cooking herself. "I like to connect with my food," she smiles. "When I examine a bunch of cilantro for freshness, inhale the citrusy burst from an orange, or cut green-pepper juliennes, I am not only taking pleasure from it, but also enriching it with my love." Who can argue with that?

Chhhannnggg!

Tiny mustard seeds descend into a pool of hot clarified butter, making a sound like raindrops pelting a tin roof. While they pop and crackle in the pan, a pinch of asafetida, a strongly aromatic spice, joins them. The air fills with fragrance. Moments later, the cumin seeds dive in, followed by dried fenugreek leaves, turmeric, coriander, cayenne, salt, and finally a cup of diced fresh vegetables.

A few hours later upon returning from school, I fling my satchel on a chair and bend over the sizzling wok to inhale the incredible aroma. How inviting they look — those potatoes, cauliflower florets, and peas — wrapped in their glistening coat of bright red pepper flakes, sun-yellow turmeric, and black mustard seeds! When they're done, Mom sprinkles them with freshly chopped cilantro leaves.

We settle eagerly on the *chatai* (straw mat) on the kitchen floor. One by one, whole wheat chapatis (Indian bread) are lifted hot off the griddle, smeared with ghee, and delivered to our waiting plates. Accompanied by sweet-and-sour mango chutney and tall glasses of cool homemade *lassi* (yogurt drink), such spicy veggies and ladelfuls of lentils are featured on our lunch menu all summer.

ayurvedic nutrition: naturally healthy

It's time to tell you why I am rhapsodizing about my eating routine. My family's food tradition epitomizes the Ayurvedic philosophy of nutrition. That is:

1. Eat a wholesome vegetarian meal. According to Ayurvedic beliefs, food should be a pure, positive input. If it is derived by taking a life, it loses its enlivening qualities. The Ayurvedic belief is that meat is *tamasic* — carrying the negative emotions of terror, panic, and helplessness that an animal experiences while being slaughtered. Thus, such tamasic foods can give rise to

feelings of dullness, depression, and aggression. But if you cannot give up meat, read the next chapter for recommendations on when and how to eat it.

2. When you set out to balance your meals, look to harmonize flavors — not balance nutrients. The reason? Ayurvedic living means listening to your body, and the body does not understand the language of carbohydrates and proteins. It responds to the scent of lemon, the sight of green peppers, the taste of curry.

Does this mean that a vaidya will encourage you to eat chips, desserts, and whatever else you like with abandon? Of course not. The Ayurvedic encouragement to "give your body foods it likes" assumes that your body will ask for foods that nourish it. If your physiology is in balance, this will happen naturally. But more about that in a moment.

How vital a role does food play in the Ayurvedic system? The clue lies in a recent remark one of my friends made. I coaxed her to consult a vaidya for a long-standing problem of insomnia. Upon her return she phoned me, sounding a little doubtful: "Well, I've come back with a grocery list!" I told her she had hit the nail right on the head. To the vaidya, food is medicine!

Ayurvedic healers follow this elementary logic: food and drink are substances that you physically, consciously put inside your body. Your body's most minute channels — its tissues and every one of its trillions of cells —

assimilate this intake, proving in a very basic sense that "you are what you eat." If what you eat is not healthy, you cannot be healthy. That is why food should form the foundation of the healing process. Ancient Ayurvedic texts go so far as to say *"Anna Bramha,"* or "food is a form of God."

To a first-timer, a vaidya's food guidelines can be somewhat puzzling. The vaidya doesn't say "eat more protein" or "avoid sodium," but instead reels off a seemingly random list of foods to choose and those to avoid. To a person suffering skin inflammation, for example, the vaidya may say "eat more fresh cheese, broccoli, and pears, but avoid garlic, mayonnaise, vinegar, and ketchup."

What is the reasoning here?

By making changes in the contents of your platter, the vaidya is trying to restore harmony among your doshas. The dietary recommendations might initially seem tough — even impossible — to follow. But the vaidya knows that, if followed for some time, these "tough" changes will receive support from your body's own intelligence.

I know of a fifteen-year-old who, when asked by a vaidya to eat brussels sprouts, shot back with "What's that?" But thanks to a mother who was willing to place her trust in the vaidya's methods, the boy had to follow the recommended diet. One month later, he reported a surprising change in his eating habits: "I find myself wanting more brussels sprouts — and I can't imagine how I ever ate ketchup!" To the vaidya, this was no surprise. It was a corroboration of a truth that our wise ancestors discovered over centuries of observation.

That truth is simple: your current health problem or "disorder" is a result of your body's innate intelligence being compromised. In Ayurveda, there is an interesting term for this: *pragya aparadh* (*pragya* means "intellect," and *aparadh* means "mistake" — thus, "a mistake of the intellect"). When the intellect commits a mistake, the taste buds that should naturally want sweet foods, for example, start craving pungent ones.

the six tastes

To understand this concept fully, let us begin with the basics of Ayurvedic nutrition by talking about the six tastes. According to Ayurveda, every grain, fruit, vegetable, or beverage on earth — whether natural or manufactured — has one or more of six basic tastes. The Sanskrit term for taste is *rasa*, and these six rasas are:

1. madhura: sweet
2. lavana: salty
3. amla: sour
4. katu: bitter
5. tikta: pungent
6. kashaya: astringent

Further, each taste represents the qualities of one or more elements of nature, and hence has the power to increase or decrease the presence of the corresponding dosha in your system. In the beginning, this can seem confusing. But let me remind you that every single Ayurvedic theory is based on direct observation of life — and that is far easier to understand than some of today's complex scientific findings!

So think about it for a moment, and the picture will start to clear. Let's take the sweet taste. In Ayurveda, the sweet taste is believed to build those tissues that are composed of the earth and water elements. Therefore, sweet foods increase the kapha dosha. Now, if you have an irrepressible sweet tooth the kapha dosha can be aggravated, causing toxic buildup. When that happens, you would be advised to increase your intake of bitter, pungent, and astringent foods — all of which decrease kapha. Foods that contain carbohydrates, sugars, fats, and amino acids belong to the "sweet" category.

Similarly, salty, sour (acidic), and pungent foods are seen to have the "heating" qualities of fire. Therefore, they speed up the metabolic process, thus increasing pitta. Take the pungent taste, for instance. Peppers are pungent — and fiery. Therefore, peppers are likely to increase pitta. And we already know that pitta-dominated people need fewer heat-producing and more cooling elements in their life. Aggravated pitta is countered by eating more sweet foods with cooling properties.

Finally, pungent, bitter, and astringent foods send the vata dosha spiraling upward. Besides foods like bitter greens and certain gourds, the bitter taste is also found in certain herbs, such as aloe vera and goldenseal. A cooling taste, it is particularly healing to those who are dominated by the pitta dosha. In moderate amounts, bitter foods are said to detoxify and cleanse the body and mind.

All hot and spicy foods belong to the "pungent" category. Ayurvedic healers believe such foods stimulate the digestion, improve appetite, and help flush out toxins. Astringent foods have a drying and firming quality. Their dry nature counteracts the phlegmatic quality of kapha, therefore, such foods are said to have a decongesting, diuretic, and analgesic effect. Volatile oils, alkaloids, and tannins in foods such as lemon oil, tomatoes, peppers, and tea belong to these categories. They penetrate the body's tiniest channels with ease, increasing movement of waste and nutrients across your system. While this can be a good thing, too much activity in the body also creates imbalance. A disturbed vata, therefore, benefits by eating warm, salty, sweet, and sour foods.

When the doshas are perfectly balanced in your physiology, you naturally lean toward the taste groups that are beneficial to you. For example, a kapha-dominated person with doshas in balance will prefer spicy curry to rich chocolate pastry. But if that person's kapha dosha is aggravated, the intellect will commit a mistake, causing a craving for pastry and further aggravating the kapha dosha. The result is lethargy — and obesity. In the case of the fifteen-year-old boy, the vaidya prescribed a diet that led his system to ask for pitta-reducing flavors.

Whatever your dosha type, if you consider yourself to be in fairly good health, all you need to do is try to get all six tastes on your plate every time you eat. "What?" I can hear you protest, "six tastes? When I barely manage to get one taste in each meal?! And when I have no clue what 'astringent' really means?"

Relax. Here are three facts about the six tastes that are sure to make you happy:

1. There is a wide variety of foods and drinks in each category. If the vaidya has told to you get more "sweet" flavors in your food, for example, you need not tear your hair out trying to think of daily dessert ideas. In Ayurveda, foods like milk, wheat, rice, bread, and potatoes are also included in the "sweet" category. Similarly, astringent foods are not exotic wild berries. They are easily found on your supermarket shelves; beans, legumes, and leafy vegetables all have the astringent taste.

Here is a more complete list of basic foods for each category:

- Sweet: rice, milk, wheat, butter, barley, pasta, potatoes, and sweet potatoes; most legumes, such as beans, lentils, and peas; sweet fruits such as dates, figs, pears, and mangoes; sugar in any form — except honey, which is also astringent.
- Salty: any foods that contain salt, especially salt-heavy foods like pickles and chips.
- Sour: citrus fruits such as oranges, limes, and lemons; also cheese, yogurt, tomatoes, sour cream, whey, vinegar, soy sauce, sour cabbage, and wine.
- Bitter: turmeric, eggplant, zucchini, fenugreek, and leafy greens.
- Pungent: spices such as black pepper, mustard,

cumin, garlic, ginger, cayenne, and other chilies;
radishes.

- Astringent: beans, lentils, walnuts, hazelnuts,
  honey, sprouts, lettuce, rhubarb, most raw vegetables, pomegranates, apples, berries, persim-
  mons, cashews, and unripe fruits.

2. Often, a single dish will supply you with more
   than one taste. Easy-to-make condiments like
   chutneys can sometimes give you all six. For
   some simple multi-flavored ideas, see the recipes
   in chapter 9.
3. Getting all six tastes does not mean having to
   make sure you get equal amounts of each flavor.
   Just a hint of the less common tastes (astringent
   or bitter) should suffice at any given meal. The
   quantities, of course, will also depend on what
   doshas you are trying to balance — and the
   vaidya is your best guide on these proportions.

the ayurvedic "no" list

Getting the six rasas on your plate is only a small part of
the Ayurvedic recommendations. The ancient texts list a
wide range of foods to avoid — whatever your dosha
type and whatever your state of health. Here are some
basic no-nos:

- Fermented, canned, and frozen foods. These are
  devoid of natural life force, or prana.
- Microwaved foods. Cooking in the microwave

oven does not involve conventional heat — and food cooked without agni is, to the Ayurvedic way of thinking, lacking in prana. Microwave cooking is also believed to confuse the chemistry of foods, changing their innate qualities. If you cannot do without the microwave, remember that the longer you cook food in there the more goodness it is going to lose.

- Leftovers. These are heavy, hard to digest, and ama-causing. Leftover food gradually changes in chemistry, losing its prana, or life force.

- Processed foods. This category includes yeast-based foods, like most yeast-based breads and pizza dough, that are not natural and hence cause ama buildup. If you cannot give up yeast-fermented bread, the next best thing is to also eat plenty of freshly kneaded and cooked bread.

- Mushrooms. These are not really a vegetable but a fungus, and Ayurvedic teaching advises against eating fungus of any kind.

- Genetically engineered foods. Interference with the basic structure of foods saps them of their natural intelligence, rendering them undesirable — even unsafe.

choosing foods the ayurvedic way

Another interesting aspect of Ayurvedic nutrition is that it weighs the benefits of food from several angles. You might not generally think about these things, but there are several factors that determine the way a food will affect you. Here are some basic questions to ask:

1. Is the food suited to you? Ayurveda attributes specific qualities to each vegetable, fruit, spice, and herb grown on the planet. These qualities are called *gunas*. Cinnamon, for instance, is considered a "hot" spice, while cardamom is "cool." Again, peas are sweet and broccoli is bitter. Though you can slowly develop an understanding of the various spices and their properties on your own, it can admittedly be confusing in the beginning. The best way to start is to refer to the dosha-wise food charts in the appendix. If you are a kapha personality, the chart will suggest some hot and pungent foods, while for pitta there is a list of sweet and mild flavors.

2. Is the combination of foods right? According to Ayurvedic wisdom, while some food substances may be beneficial on their own, they can be toxin producing if combined in a single meal. This is because each food has a unique energy, taste, quality, and aftereffect — and hence requires a different amount of digestive fire, or agni, to digest. Therefore, combining raw and cooked foods can tax the agni. Similarly, eating fruits and proteins in the same meal interferes with sugar metabolism; fruit sugar is digested with ease, while starch takes

longer — thus resulting in the formation of toxic ama. Drinking milk soon after having a glass of juice or a bowl of yogurt can curdle the milk in the stomach, forcing the digestive system to work harder.

3. How does the food change when processed? Take the example of milk. Cold milk, straight from the refrigerator, is difficult to digest. But boiled and cooled milk, taken with a pinch of nutmeg, is lighter and a natural tranquilizer. Similarly, the properties of most foods change with the way they are processed. In general, raw foods require more agni to digest, so they stay in the stomach longer. Therefore, the Ayurvedic preference is for cooked foods over raw. Lightly cooked and mildly spiced foods are considered the most beneficial. While it is true that some nutrients are lost in cooking, that loss is compensated for by the lightness of the food. If you use a healthy cooking technique, such as sautéing, steaming, or roasting, you will be able to retain essential nutrients.

4. Is the food compatible with your location? Within the same country, there are different climate zones and therefore different ways in which our bodies respond to foods. If you've recently moved from a cold, wet place to a desert region, you will need more moist, sweet, and oily foods such as carrots, zucchini, beets, cilantro, cumin, ghee, sesame oil, and light

beans. This is because the desert environment is dominated by the dry vata dosha. Clarified butter, or ghee, lubricates and nurtures the body from the inside, so it is especially good for people living in desert lands. In the same way, coastal towns and green belts have their own seasonal doshas and food requirements.

5. Is the quantity right? Each of us has a certain capacity, beyond which the system has to struggle to digest food. Typically, a pitta type of person can eat large amounts of food and digest it without trouble. A vata person has a rather irregular appetite, while a kapha-type person, whose digestion is somewhat sluggish, is satisfied with smaller amounts of food. Your appetite and capacity will depend on both your prakriti, or original constitution, and your vikriti, or current dosha state. This capacity is known in Ayurveda as your unique *matra.* Consuming much more or less than your ideal matra will cause an imbalance in your digestive system, so get a feeling for your capacity and try to eat accordingly. Whatever your dosha type, the Ayurvedic recommendation is to leave one-quarter of your stomach empty so as not to put a strain on the digestive fire. How do you know when your stomach is "three-fourths full and one-fourth empty?" Go by feel. Chew every bite well. When you have eaten enough to feel satisfied, but not full or stuffed, put your fork down.

Avoid second helpings. Don't read or watch television while eating because these activities prevent you from eating mindfully, and can cause you to overeat. By not loading your stomach with food, you help your digestive juices work more efficiently. This keeps undigested food — and hence ama — from piling up in your system, staving off the possibility of disease.

As with understanding the intricacies of your doshas, don't worry too much about balancing every aspect of the food you eat. For one thing, it is not practical, and for another, it is not necessary. To help you make good food choices with minimum fuss, I've coined two acronyms. The next time you go grocery shopping, ask yourself: "Is this food both FOR and YUP?"

FOR: Fresh and Organic.

YUP: suited to Your Unique Personality.

If the food meets both criteria, take it home.

This, then, is a basic introduction to the Ayurvedic way of nutrition. As you go along, however, you will realize that you have several questions about individual foods. For instance, "Which vegetables should I favor?" "Is yogurt good for me?" "If raw foods are hard to digest, then what about salad?" And so on.

Turn the page, and you'll find answers to these and several other basic concerns.

the when-what-how-
and-why of food

Laughter is brightest where food is best.

— Irish proverb

If you were setting out to eat a "balanced diet" based on the USDA's food pyramid, you would easily know how much to eat of what, based on your age, level of activity, and gender. But according to Ayurvedic belief, your dietary needs are so unique that such a standardized guide would not work.

Also, in Ayurveda choosing what to eat depends on more factors than just what suits your dosha type. You have to think of such complex and ever-changing factors as season, location, blend of tastes, and an ingredient's own qualities. While this makes a lot of sense, it can also make the Ayurvedic way of nutrition seem more difficult to follow.

The good news is that there are dozens of basic nutrition rules that everyone can follow, and in this chapter I will give you a quick list of these rules. Here you will find both general and specific guidelines on the fine art of choosing, preparing, and consuming your food.

Before you start reading these guidelines, I'd like to remind you that Ayurvedic nutrition is not so much about sticking to lists and quantities as it is about making intuitive and intelligent food choices.

ayurvedic nutrition basics

Here are the guidelines that will make it easier for you to eat Ayurvedically:

Eat Less Meat

As I mentioned earlier, according to Ayurveda meat is a tamasic food — one that carries the negative emotions of terror, panic, and helplessness that an animal experiences while being slaughtered. The Ayurvedic belief is that such tamasic foods can give rise to feelings of dullness, depression, and aggression. However, a great many people grow up eating meat and cannot think of giving it up. If you're one of them, try eating meat-based meals mostly at lunch, when your agni is strong enough to digest them well. Simultaneously, start making friends with the flavor-intensive world of vegetables. In Ayurveda, a vegetarian diet is considered pure, light, and *ojas* enhancing — ojas being the essential energy of the immune system.

Never "Grab" a Meal

Ayurvedic sages said *"Aaharah Praanah,"* which means "food is life." Give food the respect it deserves. Choose your ingredients with care and cook them with pleasure. Sit down to your meal, even if it is only an apple. Bring positive thoughts to the dining table and eat in the company of people who make you happy. Instead of watching television or reading a book with your meal, take in the sight, smell, texture, and flavor of your food.

It's not that we don't appreciate the value of leisurely dining. For your wedding anniversary, you don't grab a burger; you reserve a corner table at a romantic restaurant. Memories of such special occasions linger a long time; you remember the texture of every morsel, the restful ambiance, the warmth of candlelight and conversation. Such food is satisfying and nourishing in numerous ways. The Ayurvedic sages would approve if you converted your dining room into a place where every meal is a celebration.

Just Bought, Served Hot

Eat warm, freshly cooked food as often as you can. Fresh foods are rich in prana, or life force. That is why produce from a farmers' market tastes far superior to store-bought fruits and vegetables. Here is the best way to cook your vegetables:

- Heat ghee (clarified butter) to a moderate temperature, then add spices to it. This quick procedure releases the volatile oils of the spices into the ghee, drawing out their therapeutic qualities.
- Once the spices begin to sizzle in the ghee, add freshly chopped vegetables. The spices will thus be fully assimilated with your veggies, lending them flavor, aroma, color, and healing goodness.
- Simmer the vegetables on a low flame until they are just done, not mushy. To prevent burning, add a few spoonfuls of water.

As an alternative to using this method, you can also stir-fry, boil, grill, or steam your foods for maximum nutrition benefits.

Even at work, you can enjoy a hot meal if you invest in a stainless-steel thermos to hold warm foods. In the morning, you could pour some fresh-cooked vegetables and legumes into the container and carry this meal to work along with fresh whole-grain bread. Another good cooking tool is a slow cooker, which you can set up in your office kitchenette. Using this cooker, you can start a hearty soup as soon as you get to work, and enjoy it hot and delicious by lunchtime.

Clean Plate, Clean Slate

Ayurvedic healers have always advocated eating foods that are closely linked to the earth and alive with nature's own intelligence. Obviously, leftovers don't qualify for this category. Not only does leftover food gradually lose its prana, but it is also difficult to digest. Foods like chutneys can be cooked and stored in the refrigerator for weeks, but ideally even these should be made fresh in small amounts each time.

Feed Your Agni

Agni, or digestive fire, is strongest at noon and weaker at breakfast and dinner. Eat according to the strength of your agni, and your digestion will function smoothly. Don't overstuff yourself at dinner, even if that is the only meal you can eat in peace. With a little planning, you can make lunch your major meal of the day, which is what Ayurvedic wisdom recommends that you do.

Reorganize Your Pantry

For the same reason that fermented and microwaved foods are not recommended in Ayurveda, there are some other food types to stay away from. Processed, refined, and radiated foods lack any life or nutritive value. All they do is load you with calories and rob you of vitality. Why not throw them out of your kitchen and your life? Imagine your pantry shelves bursting, instead, with the goodness of such whole grains as split mung beans, whole-wheat flour, basmati rice, barley, quinoa, and amaranth. Imagine your senses being infused with the aroma and color of fresh herbs and spices like ginger, cumin, black pepper, fenugreek, coriander, and turmeric — to say nothing of their healing qualities. Visualize your refrigerator full of the freshest seasonal and organic vegetables and fruits. Of course, it is important to be realistic; you cannot achieve this transformation in one cataclysmic sweep. This process might require rethinking your budget and getting used to some new flavors. That is okay. Go slowly, but do make steady, healthful changes in the way you eat.

Discover Ghee-licious Cuisine

The Ayurvedic cooking medium of choice is ghee (clarified butter). Rich in antioxidants, ghee fights the harmful effects of free radicals. It is known to be an effective carrier of lipid-soluble nutrients; herbs and spices coated in ghee are readily absorbed by the body, thus making a healthy meal even more nutritious. What's more, ghee is so flavorful and aromatic that a little goes a long way. In fact, the benefits of ghee are so great that Ayurveda gives it the status of a *rasayana*, or preeminent healing food. You can easily make ghee at home using the recipe in chapter 9.

Fresh Ways with Salad

Now that you're stocked up and ready, let's start with salad. Salad as you know it — fresh, crunchy, raw vegetables — forms a very small part of Ayurvedic cuisine. Surprising, isn't it, when you think how much value Ayurveda places on fresh produce? But vaidyas prefer cooked food because raw vegetables require a lot of digestive fire, or agni. Therefore, Ayurvedic salads are lightly cooked. Pick your ingredients from among beans, grains, vegetables, nuts, rice, and noodles. For maximum benefit, eat them daily with lunch, when your digestive power is at its peak. Play with colors, textures, and flavors for natural balance and variety.

The Way to Eat Veggies

Warm, fresh, organic vegetables should constitute a substantial portion of your meal. Try to get at least two different vegetables at each meal, choosing those that complement each other in color, texture, and flavor. For example, carrots (which balance both vata and kapha) and broccoli (which balances pitta) make a good pair. Similarly, pitta-pleasing cauliflower and vata-friendly green beans go together well. If possible, eat one dark leafy-green vegetable such as collard, spinach, or kale every day. This will give you minerals that other vegetables do not. Furthermore, fresh moist greens release juices that hydrate the body down to its most minute channels, cleansing and refreshing you as a whole. For best results, choose your veggies based on the doshas you are trying to balance (see the "Dosha-Wise Food Guide" in the appendix).

The Protein Platoon

All beans, peas, and lentils are classified as legumes. They rank high in Ayurvedic nutrition because they're a great vegetarian source of protein. Legumes contribute an astringent taste and they strengthen body tissue, including muscle. If you're new to legumes, it will take some time to get used to digesting their protein, so introduce them gradually into your diet. Using spices such as asafetida, cumin seeds, fresh ginger, and black pepper will help you digest legumes more easily and reduce side effects such as bloating or gas. The lightest legume is mung dal, split and skinned, which you can purchase in an Asian grocery store. This quick-cooking lentil balances all three doshas.

Rice Is Nice

Here's a quick quiz: which of these grains does an Ayurvedic healer prefer — brown rice or white rice? Though brown rice has its hull and bran intact, Ayurvedic healers prefer white rice because it is easier to digest. Among white rice varieties, vaidyas say basmati is king. Long-grained and delicate, basmati rice nourishes body tissue and balances your vital energies. However, even basmati rice is not recommended daily; on its own it is a bit heavy. Those with a dominant kapha dosha should especially avoid eating rice frequently because its heavy, sweet qualities can aggravate that dosha. It is a good idea to alternate rice with other beneficial grains, such as quinoa, wheat, amaranth, and millet. Parboiled, instant, and precooked rices are definite no-nos in Ayurvedic cuisine, which considers them devoid of vital life force.

Combat Snack Attacks

You might think that Ayurveda, with its emphasis on regular mealtimes, frowns upon snacks. Not so. Snack all you like; just make sure you don't munch on tidbits until your last meal is digested. Fried snacks are devoid of prana, and hence not recommended. Recommended

Ayurvedic snacks include almonds, raisins, whole-grain bagels or sandwiches, and fresh, sweet, juicy fruit such as pears or plums.

Rethink the Way You Drink

Imagine that you've been looking forward to a great family evening by the fireplace in deep winter. Once a merry fire gets going and the conversation begins to flow, would you suddenly douse the logs with cold water? Of course not. But without knowing it, this is exactly what you might have been doing to the digestive fire inside you. When you start a meal with iced water or chilled soda, you are literally dousing your agni. No wonder, then, that in spite of a fresh hot meal you often feel heavy and uncomfortable. When you start with a cold drink and then eat a piping hot meal, you throw your stomach's digestive mechanism out of gear, inviting cramps and bloating. Solution: take all your drinks at room temperature. This simple change in the way you drink beverages will make a dramatic difference in the way you digest your meals.

Summer Coolers

Kick-start your digestion with an instant yogurt drink called *lassi* before or during your lunch (you'll find the recipe in chapter 9). Fresh and light, this delicious liquid is rich in digestion-friendly lactobacilli. Because it is a diluted form of yogurt, lassi benefits even pitta dosha, which is generally averse to sour foods, including yogurt. Here are some more heat-busting ideas:

- Make juice from water-rich fruits and vegetables like watermelon, cucumber, and lettuce for extra relief.
- Drink fresh coconut milk for relief from the heat.
- Make delectable cooling chutneys from herbs such as mint, cilantro, and watercress. For more thorough hydration, steep these cooling herbs in boiling water each morning, then bring them to room temperature and drink that water through the day.
- Favor cooling spices such as cardamom, coriander, and fennel in daily summer cooking.
- Use rose water or rose-petal conserve as a cooling food supplement, or add it to summer drinks.

Winter Warmers

The cold months are dominated by the vata dosha, so choose foods that are moist, warm, rich, and sweet. Make ripe, sweet fruits a part of your daily diet. Hot cream of wheat or rice cereals are a good choice for breakfast. A cup of herb tea is particularly soothing on cold afternoons. Slow-simmered soups using vegetables and grains make a hearty meal on their own. Hot stews like vegetarian Hungarian goulash, warm pasta, or mixed-vegetable pies topped with crumbled bread and cottage cheese are a perfect Ayurvedic choice for a winter lunch.

Water Relief

Drink at least seven to eight glasses of pure spring water during the day. Water performs the all-important function of sweeping away toxic ama from the body's tissues and cells, thus ensuring that your vital energies flow smoothly. For variety, add a sprig of fresh mint or a teaspoon of pure rose water to your glass occasionally. Water kept in the cellar or a cool room is about the right temperature for digestion on a hot day. If you cannot do without refrigerated water, do the next best thing: set it out for ten to fifteen minutes to reduce the chill. This might sound contradictory, but when you avoid ice-cold drinks, you'll find yourself coping much better with hot weather. My colleague, Vaidya Ramakant Mishra, belongs to a family of Raj vaidyas — physicians to India's erstwhile kings. He adds an interesting twist to drinking water: infuse the water with spice. Here are his dosha-wise recipes for preparing Spice Water:

Hydrating Vata-Balancing Water

Boil two quarts of water for five minutes. Take it off the heat and add three mint leaves, $1/2$ teaspoon fennel seed, and $1/4$ teaspoon marshmallow root. Place the water in a thermos. Sip it throughout the day at a warm, but not hot, temperature.

Cooling Pitta-Balancing Water

Boil two quarts of water for two minutes. Take it off the heat and add $1/4$ teaspoon fennel seed, two rosebuds, and one clove. Store it hot in a thermos, but before drinking it pour it into a cup and let it cool to room temperature.

Detoxifying Kapha-Balancing Water

Boil two quarts of water for five minutes. Take it off the heat and add three basil leaves, two thin slices of fresh ginger, $1/4$ teaspoon of cumin, and $1/2$ teaspoon of fennel. Place the water and spices in a thermos, and sip the water at a hot or warm temperature throughout the day.

The Fruit Route to Feeling Fine

According to Ayurveda, fruit is one of the purest foods we can eat. Fruits enhance vitality and radiance, which come from good digestion and which Ayurveda calls ojas. For variety, try dishing up fresh-fruit chutneys: berries, stone fruits, apples, peaches, apricots, and dried fruits (in India this refers to almonds, walnuts, and cashews) — pick and blend any of these you like (not including melons, which are generally not made into chutneys because they are less stable than acidic fruits and hence difficult to keep beyond the day without preservatives). You can simply blend fresh fruit with spices, or you can cook them lightly. Either way, a chutney will stimulate agni and help digestion. Like relish, you need just a teaspoon or two of chutney to enhance a meal.

Milk Manners

Ayurvedic healers consider milk an ojas-enhancing food, provided it is organic and free of bovine growth hormone. However, a vaidya would be appalled to see you take milk out of the refrigerator, pour it straight into a glass, and gulp it down. Cold milk is considered heavy and hard to digest. The best way to drink milk, according to

Ayurvedic wisdom, is to boil it and then allow it to cool to room temperature. This reduces its mucus-causing properties. Adding a pinch or two of nutmeg or cardamom to warm milk at bedtime is an excellent means of promoting restful sleep. A note of caution: milk does not combine well with every food. Be careful not to drink milk with such sour foods as yogurt, cheese, melons, or protein-rich legumes. Together they can disrupt the intensity of your agni, disturb your acid balance, and wreak havoc on your digestive system.

Make Your Own Yogurt

Yogurt is far easier to digest than milk, and it contributes valuable nutrients to a vegetarian diet. In Ayurveda, it is not recommended that you eat store-bought yogurt, which can be sour, devoid of active bacteria, and "heavy," or difficult to digest. For maximum benefit from yogurt, therefore, make your own at home.

Making yogurt is simple:

- In the evening, stir in two tablespoons of yogurt into one quart of organic whole milk (boiled and cooled to body temperature, or about 100 degrees).
- Place this mixture in a ceramic bowl or glass jar, cover it with a lid, and put it in a warm, draft-free place (the oven is a good place; keep the heat off, but switch on the light).
- Let it sit overnight. By morning, you should have fresh homemade yogurt.

Nutty Buddies

The vegetarian diet benefits greatly from nuts, which supply fiber, minerals, and vitamins. Most of the calories in nuts come from fat, but it is mainly unsaturated fat, which performs some essential functions in the body. Almonds are considered the most energizing of nuts, and walnuts are seen as natural stress-busters. Nuts are moist and heavy in nature, therefore the vata dosha is pacified by eating nuts. Pitta should take nuts in moderation, while kapha should avoid them as much as possible. Make sure the nuts you buy are fresh and in season (nuts are freshest in fall and winter) because rancid or old nuts can actually be toxic. To keep them fresh, store them in a cool, dark place for up to two months; refrigeration helps, too. You can also freeze whole, unsalted nuts for up to a year.

help for specific situations

The general guidelines I've just given you can work for everyone. Let me also talk about some specific situations.

The Holiday Season

Take care to eat an early dinner. You might find it difficult to avoid heavy meals during this time, so eat as early as you can to help the body digest the food better. If you get hungry later in the evening, comfort yourself with a light, warm soup. Another tip: suck on fresh ginger slices spiked with lemon and salt to improve digestion.

In Case of Illness

The body's digestive fires weaken during illness, so if you have a cold, flu, or fever it makes sense to eat light. At this time, you need foods that the body can assimilate with ease. Ayurvedic healers say that split yellow mung dal is a golden food for the sick. Nutritious and light, it cooks quickly and speeds healing. You can also make *khichari* — a one-dish meal that combines rice, mung dal, vegetables, turmeric, and salt cooked in ghee. The method: heat ghee; add the spices; toss in the dal, rice, and vegetables; cook in water. If you have two cups of rice/dal/vegetables, use six cups of water.

During Menstruation or Menopause

Women are advised to eat light meals at these times. You should also be especially careful to avoid caffeinated drinks, alcohol, and foods high in salt, sugar, or additives.

On Fasting

Fasting is often advised for people who have a kapha imbalance; it helps them detoxify. Once in a while, fasting benefits everyone by cleansing the system. But be gentle with yourself; don't starve. Puree some vegetables, blend some fresh juice, or stir up a soup. Give your stomach light doses of nutrition, and your fast will serve the purpose you want it to.

follow your intuition

You have no doubt noticed that, general or specific, Ayurvedic nutrition is about following your intuition and using good, common sense. It is also about getting a feel for your agni — knowing how to stoke it, pacify it, and keep it happy.

I'm sure you cannot wait to put together a healthful Ayurvedic meal. And I cannot wait to tell you how to do that!

fresh, flavorsome, fulfilling ayurvedic recipes

A good cook is like a sorceress who dispenses happiness.

— Elsa Schiapirelli

You are about to discover, in this chapter, a stunning variety of spices and herbs. Some of these are excitingly new, while some familiar ones will take on a new twist. Whatever the flavor, Ayurvedic cooking relies heavily on the alchemy of spices and herbs. Each teaspoon of healing spices, each tiny sprig of herb, adds a little more zing, a little more health to your plate — and your life.

The recipes I've provided here are mostly from India, where Ayurveda originated. But if you haven't tried the

you are not partial to its fla-
urvedic way if you:

reduce its consump-

warm meals as often as you can.
eriment with herbs and spices on your own.
Buy the best-quality ingredients, adjust proportions, and find imaginative ways to blend
Western and Indian flavors — basically, enjoy
cooking your Ayurvedic meal without forcing
yourself to like something. There's too much
spice in life for you to limit yourself!

Before starting to cook any of the dishes in this
chapter, gather all the ingredients required and read the
recipe carefully. It should not take you more than twenty-
five minutes to cook any of these dishes. You should be
able to find the lentils and spices mentioned here in most
Asian grocery stores.

ghee

Why it's good for you: Ghee is a revered cooking medium in Ayurveda. The ancient texts call
it a rasayana — a healing food that balances
body and mind, promoting longevity. Modern
research has established that ghee is an antioxidant and contains beta-carotene. Being free
of milk solids, ghee does not spoil easily.
Further, you can use it frugally in your cooking
and yet get rich aroma and flavor.

1 pound cultured, unsalted organic butter

Place butter in a medium saucepan and slowly melt over medium heat. When the butter comes to a boil, reduce the heat and simmer the butter uncovered and undisturbed for 45 to 60 minutes. As the temperature reaches the boiling point of water, the butter's water content vaporizes and the butter foams and makes tiny, sharp, crackling noises. The milk solids in the butter will slowly settle to the bottom, leaving pale golden liquid on top that you can sieve immediately into a clean glass jar. This is ghee. Ghee stays fresh for a few weeks at room temperature. You might, however, want to refrigerate it.

homemade cottage cheese (*paneer* in hindi)

Why it's good for you: Fresh homemade cheese made from organic, hormone-free whole milk is a good source of nutrition for vegetarians.

1 quart of milk (organic, whole milk)
juice of 1 lemon

On medium-high heat, bring milk to a boil in a large, heavy-bottomed pan. Add the lemon juice and reduce to heat to low. Simmer on low heat till the milk is fully curdled (the solids should be white and the liquid should turn a cloudy green). Strain the curds through cheesecloth or several layers of muslin. Now gather the cloth, tie it together, and either press it down on a large plate with a heavy weight or hang it up to drip. After about an hour, you will have a solid chunk of cottage cheese. This is paneer. Refrigerate paneer until ready to use. Serves 6.

stewed apple

Why it's good for you: Cooked apples, eaten first thing in the morning, help to create ojas, the final and most refined byproduct of digestion. Ojas contributes to enhanced vitality, strength, immunity, and overall well-being. Sweet juicy fruits are excellent cleansers; they help eliminate impurities from the body. According to Ayurveda, it is best to eat fruits first thing in the morning, thirty minutes before other breakfast items such as hot cereal.

1 organic apple
$1/4$ cup water
1 tablespoon organic raisins
1 clove

Peel and chop apple into small pieces. Place apple in a small pot and add the water. Add raisins and clove. Bring to a boil and then turn heat to low. Cook for about 20 minutes or until the fruit is of a tender consistency. Eat warm. Serves 1.

chickpea salad

Why it's good for you: Lightly cooked and spiced, chickpeas are a good source of protein. You can substitute or add beans and lentils of your choice in this recipe.

1 cup chickpeas (cooked al dente)
3 tablespoons olive oil

$^1/_4$ cup fresh basil leaves, chopped
1 tablespoon lemon juice
$^1/_8$ cup red bell pepper, thinly sliced
salt and pepper to taste

Combine all the ingredients in a medium bowl and toss well. Allow to marinate 30 minutes before serving. Serves 2.

lassi

Why it's good for you: In peak summer heat, lassi is an instant and energizing drink. Rich in friendly lactobacilli, lassi also aids digestion.

1 cup room-temperature water
$^1/_4$ cup fresh homemade yogurt
1 pinch ground ginger
1 pinch roasted and ground cumin
1 pinch ground coriander
1 pinch salt

Blend ingredients for one minute in a blender. Drink during or after meal. Serves 1.

basmati rice

Why it's good for you: In Ayurveda, basmati rice is considered to be a highly beneficial grain that balances all three doshas. However, eating even basmati rice daily can be heavy on your system. So do make rice an important part of your diet, but try not to eat it more than four times a week. Rice is believed to promote mucus production, so if your kapha dosha is dominant, lightly roast the rice before adding water for cooking to make it lighter.

1 cup basmati rice
2 cups water (or 1 3/4 cups if you have soaked the rice
    for a bit)

In a medium pan, bring the rice and water to a boil, then cover with a lid and reduce to a simmer. Don't lift the lid or stir the rice while it is cooking. Allow the rice to cook for 15 to 20 minutes, then press a grain or two between your fingers to test it. Well-done rice should not be sticky or hard, and the grains should be separate and fluffy.

A common mistake is to add cold water to rice that is already cooking. This destroys the agni of the rice and interferes with digestion. If you are adding salt, do so after the rice is fully cooked. Serves 2.

vitality-boosting yellow lentil soup

Why it's good for you: Beans and lentils constitute an important source of nutrition; they provide protein, complex carbohydrates, fiber, and vitamins. As versatile as they are tasty, members of the legume family lend themselves to use in salads, appetizers, soups, main dishes, side dishes, and even desserts. They combine deliciously with grains, vegetables, herbs, and spices, too.

Mung beans, split, with skins removed (also known as mung dal) are considered to be excellent for all three doshas. Easier to digest than most other lentils, the yellow mung dal can be eaten every day. When cooked, mung dal takes on the consistency of a thickish soup.

1 cup split yellow mung dal
3 to 3 1/2 cups water
1/2 teaspoon turmeric
a pinch of ground coriander
a pinch of ground ginger
a pinch of ground cumin
1 pound fresh organic spinach
1/2 teaspoon fresh lemon juice
a few pinches of rock salt

In a large pan, bring the mung dal, water, turmeric, coriander, ginger, and cumin to a boil. Then reduce the heat to medium-low, and cook until the dal is soft. You should have approximately 4 cups of cooked dal when done. Steam the spinach on medium-high heat for 2 to 3 minutes, then blend quickly with dal, just enough to distribute the spinach throughout the dal without turning it into liquid. Pour into serving bowls. Sprinkle with fresh lemon juice and a pinch of rock salt. Serve with rice or a chapati. Serves 4.

chapatis: griddle-cooked indian bread

Why they are good for you: Chapatis, or flat breads, contribute the sweet taste to a meal without the help of a calorie-heavy sweetener. Made from whole-wheat flour, they lubricate body tissues, enhance physical strength, and balance the vata dosha. Though initially time-consuming to make, chapatis are so delicious that you will want to eat them daily. If you feel you have a vata imbalance, eat plenty of wheat products such as bulgur, farina, couscous, semolina, pasta, and bread. People with a kapha imbalance should reduce but not totally avoid wheat, which can cause weight gain and increase mucus production.

2 cups sifted whole-wheat flour, whole-wheat pastry flour, or chapati flour (called *atta*, found at Indian grocery stores)
$1/_2$ teaspoon salt
$2/_3$ cup lukewarm water
small amount of ghee

Combine the flour and salt in a large mixing bowl and knead while gradually adding water to make a moist dough. Fold and push the dough until it stops sticking to your hands; this should take about 10 minutes. Cover the dough with a clean, damp cloth and let it rest for 30 minutes. While the dough is resting, prepare your lentils, vegetables, and salad or whatever you plan to serve with the chapatis.

Heat a cast-iron skillet or a heavy nonstick griddle on your stove at maximum heat. Meanwhile, quickly knead the dough again, then cover it again with a damp cloth. Now pull out a lemon-sized portion of the dough from underneath the cloth and shape it into a ball. Next, with a rolling pin, roll the ball out evenly into a thin circular shape (about 6" to 8" in diameter) on a floured cutting board. Repeat with another portion of the dough, always keeping the rest of it covered with the cloth. Do not stack the rolled-out chapatis or they will stick to each other. You could use wax paper to stack them, but make sure the topmost disk is also covered; the idea is to keep the dough from drying out.

To cook, place each chapati on the heated skillet one at a time. Once the chapati starts cooking, you will need to fine-tune the heat: generally, it needs to be lowered very slightly. Because stove temperatures can vary, you will arrive at the right cooking temperature for your chapatis with practice. Watch for small white bubbles to appear on the surface; this takes just about 10 seconds. Using a non-melting plastic spatula, flip the chapati and cook for 1 minute. Press lightly on the cooking chapati with a clean cloth or paper towel rolled up into a ball, and the chapati will start to fluff up and turn a mottled brown. If you have an electric stove, you will have to fluff up your chapati fully at this stage by turning it over and over, and gently rotating it on the skillet. If you have a gas stove, remove the chapati from the griddle with a pair of metal tongs and place it over a direct flame. The chapati should puff up into a ball almost immediately. Remove from heat, smear with a teaspoon of ghee, and serve hot. Making perfectly puffy chapatis takes practice, but is truly worth the effort. Makes up to 15 chapatis, depending on size you make them.

chutneys

Why chutneys are good for you: Made with the freshest of fruits, herbs, and spices, chutneys are a great way to get beneficial antioxidants in your meal. A good chutney can give you all six tastes in two teaspoonfuls: sweet, salty, sour, bitter, pungent, and astringent. Chutneys aid in digestion and add interest to a meal. Spicy chutneys bring balance to mild dishes, and sweet chutneys bring balance to spicy dishes.

cilantro chutney

2 cups fresh cilantro (leaves and tender stems), washed and roughly chopped

1 cup fresh mint leaves

1 ancho chili or other mild chili

1 teaspoon fresh minced ginger

$1/2$ teaspoon whole cumin seeds

1 tablespoon lemon juice

salt to taste

Combine all ingredients in a blender and puree to a smooth paste. Serve as an accompaniment to a meal or as a topping or spread. This chutney balances all three doshas.

cooked apple chutney

2 organic apples, peeled, cored, and chopped

$1/4$ cup raisins

$1/2$ teaspoon cinnamon

$1/2$ teaspoon ground ginger

$1/4$ teaspoon grated lemon rind

juice of $1/4$ lemon

$1/8$ teaspoon salt

1 tablespoon sugar

$1/4$ cup water

Place all ingredients in a medium pot and bring to a boil. Reduce heat and simmer uncovered for about 30 minutes, stirring occasionally.

fruit compote (dessert)

Why it's good for you: In Ayurveda, fruit is comparable to gold. It increases ojas — the essential energy that is generated by well-oiled body-mind machinery. Fruit desserts are light and help with digestion. Since the Ayurvedic practice is to eat fruit on its own, it is best to have this dessert thirty minutes after your meal.

$1/3$ cup slivered almonds

1 cup orange juice

1 cinnamon stick

$1/2$ teaspoon anise seeds

$1/2$ teaspoon grated lemon rind

1 tablespoon grated orange rind

1 pound whole apricots or frozen peach slices (thawed)

1 pound pitted Bing cherries, fresh or frozen (thawed), not canned

2 navel oranges, sliced and peeled

$1/4$ cup honey

Soak the almonds in water overnight. In a medium to large pot, add spices and citrus rinds to the orange juice. Bring to a boil, then reduce heat to medium and cook uncovered for about 5 minutes. Strain out seeds, and add fruit to the spiced orange juice. Return mixture to the cooking pot and bring to a boil. Simmer for 15 minutes. Remove from heat and allow to cool to a slightly warm temperature. Add honey, sprinkle slivered almond over fruit, and serve warm. Makes 6 to 8 servings.

appetizing ways with herbs and spices

If you have just discovered the wonders of herbs and spices but don't quite know how to savor them to the fullest, here's help. Each of the following ideas is a healthy, delicious mini-recipe. You can adjust ingredient quantities to your taste and requirement. Start with these, and you will soon find yourself thinking up many more exciting combinations.

raita

There's something about yogurt and mint; they make magic together. Make fresh yogurt at home, then whisk it until its smooth. Now stir in a grated cucumber. Float a few sprigs of finely chopped mint in this sea of flavor, dust with roasted and ground cumin seeds, and fill your senses with the incredible aroma. Add appetizing color to this dish with a pinch of paprika.

cumin rice

Cumin is one of India's star spices, praised for centuries for its digestion-friendly and detoxifying qualities. It's a versatile spice, too. Use it raw, roasted, or fried, and each time it will reward you with a different flavor and aroma. Try this simple cumin rice: Heat a tablespoon of ghee, then add a teaspoonful of cumin seeds. When the seeds splutter, add washed rice and the required quantity of water (see the recipe for basmati rice earlier on page 129).

When the rice is done, fluff it with a fork, tossing in a few sprigs of fresh chopped cilantro. If you enjoy your rice a bit tangy, squeeze a twist of lemon into the rice at this time. Bonus: lemon helps fluff out rice grains.

bouquet garni

"Bouquet garni" is a culinary term for spices and herbs tied together in a muslin cloth and steeped in a soup or stew. Once the ingredients have released their scent and digestion-promoting goodness into the dish, the muslin pack is removed. I use bay leaves, cloves, cinnamon sticks, and black peppercorns to spice up chickpeas as they boil. Try it with peas, kidney beans, and other legumes — and I am sure you will love the extra flavor they lend.

discovering ajwain

Let me tell you about ajwain, a warming and detoxifying spice. It tastes somewhat like thyme, but stronger. I find it somewhat similar to oregano, too. The best way to discover the distinct taste of ajwain, of course, is to sample it. In India, we like to spike our fritter batter with it, but if you want to avoid deep-fried foods, as Ayurveda recommends, try kneading your bread dough with half a teaspoon of ajwain seeds for an exciting new flavor.

Here's another quick and interesting way to use ajwain: Heat 2 teaspoons of ghee, then add half a teaspoon of ajwain seeds. Wait for them to sizzle, then pitch in slices of 4 medium boiled potatoes. Add salt to taste and fry on high heat for a few minutes. I like to offset the flavor of ajwain with plenty of fresh chopped cilantro leaves; this adds a nice green color, too. Toss the cilantro in the pan and mix just before serving. Eat the potatoes hot. You can sandwich them in bread for a wholesome, delicious mini-meal.

indian-style pizza

Next time you bake a pizza, try flavoring it with some Indian herbs and spices. Sprinkle chopped cilantro leaves on the toppings; they combine particularly well with roasted veggies. Add aroma with freshly roasted and ground cumin seeds. I've even tried pizza topped with herbed mashed potato. Believe me, it is luscious!

ways with cayenne

Ever noticed how cayenne pepper can make the nose run? It's releasing mucus, clearing up your channels, and thereby balancing out the kapha dosha. Black pepper, cumin, and turmeric benefit kapha, too. Fry a very small amount of ground cayenne pepper in some olive oil or ghee, then toss in your chopped vegetables for a wonderful stir-fry. Or simply pour the ghee-and-pepper garnish over soup or lentils. You'll welcome the channel-clearing warmth — doubly so if you've been suffering from clogged sinuses.

saffron rice pudding

To make rice pudding, slow cook half a cup of basmati rice with four cups of whole milk in a medium pan. When thickened to the consistency of custard, stir in sugar to taste.

When the pudding is thickened and nearly done, simmer rice pudding with a few strands of saffron. You'll get a rich orange coloring and a taste very close to divine. And saffron's bounty doesn't stop with flavor and color; it is very dosha-friendly, too. Vata, pitta, or kapha — all three doshas love it. Indian rice pudding, called *kheer*, is never quite complete without saffron and its partner, freshly crushed green cardamom.

colorful curries

If saffron is gold, turmeric is sunshine. Its brilliant yellow color is one of the most eye-catching components of an Indian spice box. I cannot imagine cooking most soups, lentils, or stews without turmeric; in India, we grow up on yellow-colored curries. Ayurvedic healers love turmeric for its benevolent properties and antibiotic qualities. My grandmother would heat ghee with turmeric, toss a clean piece of cotton in it, and tie it to a wound. It felt so instantly warm and healing — second only to a mother's kiss. Turmeric has great antioxidant properties, too. Add turmeric to ghee when stir-frying your vegetables. Enjoy the colorful, healing difference just one teaspoonful can make.

Make more magic with turmeric: combine it with white. Boiled white rice on its own can get boring, but cook it with turmeric and it takes on an appetizing golden color. Complement the yellow color with freshly chopped cilantro. Add cilantro to the rice only after it is done, otherwise I've noticed that the leaves wilt and turn brown. For parties, I stir-fry some cashew nuts in ghee and add them to the cooked yellow rice.

spiced lentils

Although lentils, such as yellow split mung, are light and tasty on their own, a little spice makes a big difference in flavor. Tiny black mustard seeds and cumin are favorite Indian garnishes for lentils. You can also roast and pound whole coriander seeds, then add them to boiled lentils of your choice. I usually sauté these spices in ghee. Try adding a handful of stir-fried spinach to split green lentils; it tastes delicious and adds even more health benefits.

tikiya with tangy chutney

Combine a small bunch of mint and cilantro in a blender, then add some rock salt to taste and half a lemon. This tangy chutney makes a great filling for shallow-fried mashed potatoes, which we call *tikiya*. Here's how to make it: Take a lemon-sized portion of mashed potato and flatten it in your palm. Place a teaspoon of the mint-cilantro filling on the disk, then roll it into a ball. Flatten the ball gently with your palm. Now heat a teaspoon of ghee or oil in a griddle or pan and place the potato ball on it. Fry on both sides until the edges are reddish brown. Enjoy this hot potato as a snack or a side dish. For extra flavor, you can mix some mashed green peas with the potatoes.

baked vegetables

In an ovenproof dish, marinate fresh vegetables for 15 to 30 minutes in a paste of 1 cup yogurt, $1/4$ teaspoon ground cumin, $1/8$ teaspoon ground cayenne pepper,

$^1/_2$ teaspoon tumeric, and salt to taste. Meanwhile, heat the oven to 450 degrees F, then slide the dish in. Within 15 minutes, you'll have a sizzling, healthful platter ready. I sometimes add fresh grated coconut to the marinade for a delicate flavor.

cottage cheese and veggies

In a medium pan, lightly stir-fry a tablespoon of olive oil, sliced bell peppers, and tomatoes cut lengthwise. Add a teaspoon of turmeric, then toss in some cubes of homemade cottage cheese (see recipe on page 127). Cook until the cottage cheese is lightly browned and the vegetables are tender. For an interesting twist to this simple dish, add a few tablespoons of boiled yellow lentils while frying the veggies.

cardamom carrots

Toss $^1/_2$ cup raw sliced carrots and 2 tablespoons raisins in lemon juice, then sprinkle with a generous pinch of freshly crushed green cardamom. Cardamom is a metabolism-revving spice with warming properties, so pitta types should take it in smaller amounts.

friendly fennel

In the Kashmir region of India, kidney beans are cooked with fennel as one of the spices. The flavor it imparts to the beans is very pleasant. As a bonus, fennel tones the digestive system. It is also said to stoke agni, or digestive fire, but not to the extent that it irritates the pitta dosha.

Housewives in the desert areas of western India make a refreshing fennel-based after-dinner mint. It is not only delicious, but very soothing to the digestive system. The recipe is easy: Roast a few teaspoons of fennel seeds on a cast-iron griddle or a nonstick pan with a pinch of turmeric, taking care not to let the seeds burn. When they release their aroma, put them in a bowl and toss them with just enough lemon juice to moisten the seeds. Munch after lunch.

turka

In southern India, most curried dishes are enlivened with a simple but aromatic *turka* (fried garnish). Heat one tablespoon of ghee, then add to it a teaspoon of mustard seeds, one halved dried red chili, and a small bunch of curry leaves (available in Indian grocery stores). When the mustard seeds begin to pop and the red chili darkens — this will happen within seconds, so be careful not to let them burn — pour the turka into your lentils, curry, or soup.

garam masala

Have you ever tried garam masala (literal translation: "hot spice")? It is an interesting Indian spice mix. Different regions of India make garam masala in different ways, but generally it contains cloves, nutmeg, mace, peppercorns, and cardamom. Garam masala is carried at most grocery stores. Usually, a small amount of garam masala is stirred into a curry or soup when it is just about done. This retains the flavors of the spices and adds zing to the dish. Ground fresh, the spices in garam masala are highly fragrant, flavorful, and appetizing.

spiced fruit dessert

Slice some organic sweet apples and pears, then toss them with slivers of fresh ginger and dried orange peel. Steep this fruit mix in a marinade of orange juice (just enough to cover the fruit) for about 10 minutes. Once the orange peel and ginger have infused the dessert with their flavors, remove them.

spice up your soups

What better way to beat winter blues than comforting the body with hot soup? This December, dish up hearty vegetable soups from time to time. Simmer them with fresh vegetables, pasta, grains, spices, and herbs.

---

gourmet tip

I hope you enjoy cooking the Ayurveda way. For hundreds of additional healthful, flavorful recipes, I recommend Miriam Hospodar's book *Heaven's Banquet: Vegetarian Cooking for Lifelong Health the Ayurveda Way* (Dutton, 1999). It's a treasure house of information and vegetarian recipes from across the globe.

Bon appetit!

be ayurveda beautiful

Beauty is a light in the heart.

— Kahlil Gibran

When I first set out to study the Ayurvedic paradigm of beauty, I half expected to encounter the sages' scorn for outer appearance. I felt almost sure that they would dismiss physical beauty as being "but skin-deep." I was pleasantly surprised.

Ancient Ayurvedic healers not only recognized the human need to look beautiful, they actually celebrated it. The evidence is sprinkled liberally in their writings, which pay homage to physical beauty, eulogizing long eyelashes, full lips, supple limbs, and soft skin. The revered sage Patanjali wrote, "Perfection of the body is beauty of form, grace, strength, compactness, and the hardness and brilliance of a diamond."

However, most such gems of timeless thought are more or less lost to the world today. The trend, instead, is to use "herbal" cosmetics and assume that there is nothing more to Ayurvedic beauty care. I know, because I did this for many years myself. Like millions of others, I tried every herbal brand name on the supermarket shelves — and spent a mini-fortune on "Ayurvedic" facials and massages.

But, of course, this was before I read what Ayurvedic practitioners really had to say about beauty. Yes, they recommend herbal creams and lotions. But more than that, they urge us to cultivate beauty the way you would grow a breathtaking rose: give it a healthy root system.

In other words, pay attention to everything you put inside your body and mind, for what you absorb is what you reflect. Don't expect the latest lotion on the market to rejuvenate your tired skin; start by eating a wholesome breakfast. Don't smear layers of concealer over under-eye bags; set your sleep routine in order. And before you spend thousands of dollars on liposuction, try banishing cellulite through a daily oil massage and a brisk walk.

Then, when you shed your dependence on salons and spas and take your beauty into your own hands, you will, in Ayurvedic terms, be threefold beautiful.

the three layers of beauty

In Ayurveda, physical charm is only the first layer of beauty. The Sanskrit word for this outer layer of beauty is *roopam*. Beyond your outer appearance lie two deeper layers:

- Inner beauty, or *gunam*, which indicates sincerity of heart, purity of thought, and honesty of action;
- Lasting beauty, or *vayastyag* (*vaya* means "age," and *tyag* means "giving up" — in this sense, "moving beyond the limits of"), which means looking young and lovely well into your mature years.

Of these, roopam is, of course, the most obvious and popular form of beauty. And why not? Wearing makeup and clothes that flatter you boost your self-image, which is important in Ayurvedic healing. But roopam should be more than just a paint job.

the road to roopam

You go to a party, and two women catch your eye. One of them is soft-spoken and graceful, smiles with her eyes, and has a glowing complexion. The other one turns heads for different reasons: her voice is loud, her attire is flashy, and her makeup is heavy. Which of these women would you call beautiful? If you had a choice, which of these women would you like to get to know better?

The simple-yet-graceful woman symbolizes roopam, for her beauty is free of the crutches of makeup and affectation; it is natural and honest. She has taken the time-tested route to beauty: being kind to her body, true to her heart, and in tune with the world around her.

Beauty Begins with Skin Care

It does not matter whether you are fair or dark; healthy skin simply looks happy. It glows.

How does your skin look right now? Dry or dewy? Scaly or smooth? Pale or pink? Don't worry if the answer is less than flattering at this moment. While it is true that your skin's health is your responsibility, it is also true that other factors — including the seasons and life's unceasing stresses — affect skin texture and health. But perhaps the most important of these factors is nature itself. In other words, your skin type is part of your prakriti — your original dosha type:

- Vata people have fine, thin, delicate, dry skin. On the plus side, they are unlikely to suffer rashes and pimples. On the minus side, their dry skin is prone to early aging and wrinkling.
- Pitta skin is warm, moist, and fair, but it is also very sensitive and prone to breakouts.
- Kapha people are blessed with well-lubricated skin that keeps them looking youthful for many

years. But excess kapha can clog pores and cause toxic buildup.

Knowing your dosha type, therefore, is the first step toward improving your skin's health. For example, a vata person's best skin-care treatment is hydration; vata skin needs lots of moisture in the form of water, oil, and rich lotions. If you're a pitta, you would benefit most from ingredients that soothe the skin — for example, milk, rose water, or cucumber. Kapha skin stays healthy when regularly cleansed to remove toxins. This dosha-based skin care is a unique, practical way of solving skin-related problems that are specific to you.

Whatever your dosha type, one thing is for sure: your skin is a living, breathing, pulsating organ. It is sensitive to outer stimuli, such as pleasure, pain, and heat. New scientific evidence corroborates the Ayurvedic theory that your skin actually "drinks" what you apply on the surface — even water. Think, then, what happens when it drinks harsh chemicals that penetrate its delicate inner layers and mingle with the bloodstream.

The Ayurvedic advice is to feed your skin the way you would feed your body: never apply anything to your skin that you would not eat. In practical terms, this means making sure that you use only skin-care products that are perfectly pH-balanced, free of toxic chemicals, and therefore safe to apply.

While you can certainly find genuine herbal products in stores, I invite you to discover some stellar beauty ingredients right inside your kitchen. Turmeric, milk, yogurt, peaches, honey, almonds — let these be your cosmetics. Play with face packs. Try making your own; they're safe, inexpensive, and fun to make. They will purify your skin and make it radiant as a dewy rose.

To help you figure out the best ingredients for your type of skin, I asked my vaidya, Ramakant Mishra of Maharishi Ayurveda, a company that manufactures and distributes premium Ayurvedic formulations, to provide some easy skin-cleansing face packs you can make at home. Here are the recipes he created:

Cleansing Masks
for dry skin

    2 teaspoons quick-cooking oats
    $1/4$ teaspoon almond powder
    $1/4$ teaspoon grated orange peel
    $1/4$ teaspoon lavender-flower powder (available in
        good natural health stores)
    2 tablespoons yogurt

Stir all the ingredients together and apply the mixture gently to your face with your fingertips. Let the mask set on your skin. Then, using light pressure, flake the mask off into the sink. If the mask feels too sticky, use warm water to rinse. Dab your face with a soft towel and apply a good moisturizer.

Instant oatmeal is an excellent skin exfoliant; oats counteract daily sun damage and replenish the skin with vitamins B and E. Orange peel balances the pH level of the skin and softens it. Almond powder is a protein-packed exfoliant. Yogurt contains friendly lactobacilli that pacify an aggravated pitta. And the healing aroma of lavender powder makes this a soothing, pleasant mask.

for oily skin

1 tablespoon yogurt
1 teaspoon toasted wheat bran
$1/4$ teaspoon almond powder
$1/2$ teaspoon grated orange peel
1 teaspoon lemon juice

Mix and apply the mask in the same manner as for the Dry Skin Mask.

Wheat bran is a very efficient cleanser, coaxing out grime with ease. Combined with cooling yogurt, it makes a gentle exfoliant. The vitamin C in lemon juice promotes cleansing activity.

for sensitive skin

Make the same mask as for dry skin, but substitute whole raw (uncooked) milk for yogurt, and use rose-petal powder instead of grated orange peel. In Ayurveda, the rose is held in high regard; it is soothing, healing, and extremely nourishing.

Caring for the Rest of You

This safe, natural beauty care, should, of course, not be limited to skin cleansers and moisturizers. Whatever other body-care products you use — shampoos, hair conditioners, makeup — be sure they are gentle and nourishing, not enemies in disguise.

But wait — there is much more to roopam than just

cosmetic care. If you imagine your body to be a house, then roopam is only the facade. Obviously, painting the house from the outside is no help if the interiors are in ruin. In other words, no amount of moisturizer or nail polish can make you look good if your digestion is upset and your mouth feels stale. Conversely, if your vital systems are in great working order, your face and your skin will reflect that inner glow.

The way to achieve true roopam, therefore, is to nurture your body through good diet. This does more than help metabolism. It suffuses you with ojas — that certain something that beautiful people radiate, without assistance from cosmetics.

Remember, you produce ojas in inverse proportion to ama. The lower your body's ama, or toxin content, the higher your personality's ojas, or radiance quotient, and vice versa. So keep toxin elimination as a priority in your list of beauty to-dos. Two easy, pleasurable ways to shed toxins and acquire ojas are daily self-massage and regular exercise.

The Magic of Massage

Daily self-massage is called *abhyanga*. All it takes is fifteen minutes, and look at the benefits you get:

- When you massage your body, you lavish it not only with lubricant, but also with love. Touch is a basic human need, and through massage you give yourself a healing touch.

- Most of the day, your skin suffers in silence,

feeling dry, dull, and neglected. A regular oil massage gives it much-needed sheen, moisture, and warmth.

- No matter what your dosha type, massage restores your balance and makes you feel relaxed.

- Massage is an almost instant healer; the oils penetrate deep into body tissues within seconds, nourishing you from within.

- Massage is an excellent way to detoxify. The rubbing and stroking actions dislodge accumulated toxins, which then move out of the body through the digestive system.

- In the long run, regular massage maintains the youthfulness of skin, keeping it lustrous and healthy throughout your life.

Mmm – Massage: How to Give Yourself a Refreshing Rubdown

Begin by heating your massage oil to purify it (see the appendix for guidance in selecting the best oil for your dosha type). Called *curing*, this process makes the oil easier to absorb and enhances its antioxidant qualities. To cure your oil, pour a quart — which should last you about two weeks — into a pan and bring it to a boil on a low flame. Then drop a tiny bit of water into the oil. If you hear an instant "pop," your oil is cured. (If there is no "pop," keep heating until you hear one.) After the "pop" sound, take the oil off the stove. Cool the oil a bit, then pour it into an easy-squeeze, flip-top bottle. Take some simple precautions while curing the oil: do not leave it unattended, do not heat it on a high flame, only drop a tiny bit of water to test whether the oil has cured to avoid splattering, and do not pour it into a bottle while it's hot.

Now to the massage itself. Warm oil penetrates tissues faster and feels good on your skin. Therefore, just before massaging yourself, reheat the oil by running the bottle under the hot water tap for a minute or two — or, if you have the time, heat a small amount of oil in a pan. When you are ready, remove all your clothing and jewelry and sit down on an old towel so you won't make a mess.

Start at the top: massage your head first. Pour a small quantity of oil into your cupped palm and raise it to your scalp. Then, swiftly opening your palm, let the oil kiss the top of your head. This is your introduction to bliss. Now move your palm in circles, rubbing the oil gently but thoroughly all over your head. Part your hair from time to time so that the oil seeps right into your scalp. Ayurvedic healers recommend spending maximum time on head massage, and for good reason. According to Ayurveda, there are 107 vital points just beneath the skin. Called *marmas*, they are believed to be connecting points between the mind and the body. Thirty-seven of these marma points are located in the head and neck area. This is what makes head massage so relaxing.

After massaging your head, move down to your face, the outer part of your ears, your neck (both front and back), your shoulders, and your upper back. Be sure to rub gently on your face. Also, you will find that massaging your ears feels particularly nice.

Now dab some oil down the length of your arms, then rub the oil into your arms using long back-and-forth strokes. Rub around your elbows and knuckles in a circular motion, applying gentle pressure.

Rub some more oil up and down your chest, massaging your breasts in gentle circular strokes. When you reach your abdomen, make sure your strokes are in a clockwise motion, for that is the direction in which your large intestine moves.

Massage your legs in much the same manner as you did your arms: back and forth along the bones, with circular strokes around your knees and ankles. Lavish some time on your feet; they are often the most neglected part of our anatomy.

By now, you should be experiencing a unique feeling: that of being deliciously rested and wonderfully refreshed. You might want to allow the oil to soak into your pores for a while, and that is an excellent idea.

Now you can gently wipe excess oil from your body (to avoid clogging your drain) using your old towel. Then, using a mild, oil-based vegetable or herbal soap, wash the oil away in a warm shower. If you have the time, a warm bath is even more relaxing.

How much time should you spend on your daily massage? Ayurvedic physicians recommend ten to fifteen minutes of daily oil massage for maximum benefit. If you are rushed for time, give it five minutes, which is better than skipping it altogether.

Walk Those Toxins Off

There is a good reason why athletes and cyclists never suffer from cellulite: they keep moving, so ama never gets a chance to build up inside them. But most of us would not want to — and cannot hope to — do such strenuous exercise. The good news is that Ayurveda does not demand that you work out so hard. Ayurvedic wisdom favors walking as a form of exercise because it is nonstrenuous and calming. Moreover, unlike several other forms of exercise, walking gives your body a complete workout, improving circulation and eliminating ama without putting strain on any one group of muscles.

The three dosha types have different exercise requirements, and walking fulfills all these needs. For example:

- Vata people, being energetic but restless, will plunge readily into exercise but tire quickly. For such people, a brief brisk walk is the ideal solution.
- Pitta people, who are so dynamic and intense that they tend to overexert themselves, find walking a moderate alternative to aggressive competitive sports.
- Kapha people, by nature laid-back and lethargic, enjoy the easy pace of walking.

a beautiful mind: gunam

Good digestion, sparkling eyes, shining hair — yes, these are indicators of beauty. And yet they are meaningless if your favorite expression is a scowl, or your dominant mood blue.

Of course, it is stress that causes most of our scowls and blue moods. But I recently read somewhere that "Life is one percent what happens to you, and ninety-nine percent how you respond to it." Ayurveda embraces this truth; change the way you respond to life's demands, and you will find inner beauty, or gunam.

The best place to begin your quest for gunam is, again, to refer to your basic nature. This means turning to your dosha types once again — but this time to doshas with a difference. You might be surprised to learn that, just as you have three physical doshas (vata, pitta, and kapha), there are three doshas of the mind. Vaidyas call these doshas *gunas,* or qualities. These are: *rajas, tamas,* and *sattva.*

The qualities of these behavioral doshas do not correspond to those of their physical counterparts — vata, pitta, and kapha. That is, rajasic behavior doesn't have vata qualities, tamas is not the mental aspect of pitta, and sattva doesn't have kapha qualities. Rajas, tamas, and sattva have their own distinct qualities, which will be clear from the following simple example.

Three men are traveling together in a train when their compartment catches fire. Watch their reactions:

- The first person has a dynamic nature, which spurs him to take immediate action; he starts hunting for the nearest fire extinguisher or exit. Such people are said to have a rajasic mind, which naturally relies on action.

- The second person panics, then faints. Such people, whose minds are dull, weak, or tamasic in nature, find themselves unable to act or react in a manner suited to the needs of a situation.

- The third person is blessed with a sattvic mind. Being calm and steady, he takes a moment to analyze the situation and acts only after weighing the possibilities and determining the right response to the situation.

All of us possess all three gunas, but some of us have more rajas, others more tamas, and, perhaps fewer of us, more sattva in our nature. But this doesn't mean that we cannot change the proportion of these gunas in us. From the example above, it is obvious that sattva is the highest guna, worthy of cultivation. You can increase your sattva quotient if you set yourself some day-to-day behavior guidelines:

- Indulge in activities that bring you pleasure. When the mind is happy in itself, it wants to spread that joy among others.

- Conversely, do not indulge in activities that build up toxic thoughts and feelings. Don't watch violent movies or read crime fiction in excess. Don't harbor a grudge.

- Take time to do a good deed: make a child smile, spend time with an aged person, plant hope in an unhappy heart.

- Take a balanced approach to your relationships; love, but don't nag or cling. Give without expecting in return.

- Treat yourself gently. Don't set yourself impossible deadlines and goals. Remember, when you look at life through the glasses of materialism, you don't get the true picture.
- Let there be moderation in every aspect of your life, be it diet, sleep, sex, exercise, work, or ambition.

These are habits that cannot be cultivated overnight. But if you are mindful of their sattva-enhancing value, you can make positive changes in your day-to-day behavior. And that is a great way to begin.

lasting beauty: vayastyag

According to Ayurveda, true beauty defies chronology. It beats back the forces of stress and refuses to age socially or psychologically. Such beauty is vayastyag, and it comes when there is perfect *samanvaya,* or balance, between both roopam and gunam. In this state of balance, a person achieves *sat chit ananda,* or purity of soul and total bliss, which the Vedas say is the definition of complete beauty.

Believe Yourself Beautiful

Perhaps one of the biggest reasons people fail to look beautiful is that they don't feel beautiful. Blame it on the models and movie stars who represent beauty in these times, but the fact remains: a society's ideals of beauty can be damaging to a person with a less-than-perfect figure or features.

Ayurveda considers this negative self-image a serious

enemy of beauty. Like unreasonable food cravings, this negative self-perception is also seen as a mistake of the intellect, or pragya aparadh. Because your body hears everything you think, the damage from this condition eats into your very consciousness and shows up on your face.

If this is how you have been feeling, start healing yourself by making positive affirmations to yourself every day. For example:

I am one with nature, and nature is beautiful. My body and mind are like a temple; I won't defile them with chemical-laden cosmetics, life-less foods, or toxic thoughts. I'll be true to myself and to those I love, for I am more than roopam (outer beauty), I am gunam — beautiful from the inside.

Say these words out loud to yourself once a day, and watch the difference they make. What's more, these simple words put you in direct contact with yourself — something Ayurveda deeply encourages.

The most revered Ayurvedic text, *Charaka Samhita*, suggests a fun way to look and feel young as long as you live: simply seek the company of those who are young at heart. Their influence will bring laughter and optimism into your life, bestowing you with youth's carefree spirit.

This, then, is the essence of Ayurvedic beauty: a healthy mix of good diet, sattva-enriching lifestyle, and positive thinking. Set aside that antiwrinkle cream and drink some water instead. Whistle on your way to work. Smile. You will look gorgeous and feel beautiful — lit from within.

massage dos and donts

- DO choose an oil that will balance your individual dosha type. Although sesame oil benefits all three doshas, the cooling quality of coconut oil is highly beneficial for pitta skin. Vata skin will love the rich, moist quality of almond oil. Kapha skin, being naturally moist, needs smaller amounts of oil; sesame oil is ideal for kapha.
- DO use cold-pressed, chemical-free, organic oils.
- DO massage with warm oil. It feels and penetrates better.
- DO leave the oil on your skin for up to forty-five minutes. This helps the oil heal and nourish tissue better.
- DO follow up your massage with a warm bath or shower.
- DO relax between applying the oil and taking a shower. Listen to music, read a book, or simply think happy thoughts.
- DON'T skip your post-massage shower; oil retained on the skin too long can clog channels.
- DON'T use harsh soap after your massage; the detergent will leach the oil from your pores. Use a mild oil-based herbal soap. If your skin is not very sensitive, you can also use barley or chickpea flour to gently lift the oil — and with it, dead cells — from the surface of your skin.

simply stress-free

Take rest; a field that has rested gives a bountiful crop.

— Ovid

Monday, 9:30 A.M. Traffic lights flash on the streets of Los Angeles. Horns blare. Cars streak along the freeway. Golden sunlight bounces off the waves of the Pacific, but no one has the time to stop and gaze. Life is on autopilot.

Waiting in the reception area of a seaside office building, thirty-five-year-old Meryl pulls at her cheek to calm a persistent twitch. Minutes later, she sits across from a cheerful man who nods understandingly as her story comes tumbling forth.

That man, a vaidya, counsels dozens of angst-ridden men and women every day. It does not surprise or alarm him to hear that the young woman before him seems to be suffering from every conceivable problem, from back-ache, headache, and wristache to insomnia, depression, and chronic fatigue. Ninety percent of the patients he sees have similar stories to tell. The diagnosis: burnout.

In a world increasingly addicted to instant solutions — instant coffee, instant messaging, instant trading — Meryl could have taken her pick of instant medications: tranquilizers, sedatives, soporifics. Why is she seeing a vaidya instead? Perhaps because, like millions of other people, Meryl has begun to realize that instant remedies are not worth the price you pay in side effects.

To a vaidya, the option of suppressing stress with side-effect-causing pills simply does not arise. The vaidya knows that your stress has its origins in one of three places: your body, your mind, or your spirit. The first priority is to figure out the point of origin, then recommend simple ways to set you free of stress. The advantage in this approach is that you are encouraged to become your own physician. Here is how you, too, can detect the origins of your stress.

begin with the body

The human body is one of the most intelligent, resilient structures in all of creation. The kapha dosha rules body framework, holding bones and muscles together and providing support and strength. As long as you use your body well, the kapha dosha makes sure your body performs at peak levels.

But when you tax your body beyond reasonable limits, or simply do not use it enough, you start accumulating toxic ama inside your body. And, as we have seen, the kapha dosha cannot tolerate ama at all. In particular, two of kapha's deputies, or subdoshas, are affected by physical stress:

- tarpaka kapha, which maintains moisture in such body channels as the sinuses, mouth, and eyes, and is also responsible for nourishing the five senses — sight, hearing, touch, taste, and smell;
- sleshaka kapha, which looks after the health of the joints.

Disturbed, these subdoshas start sending distress signals, which, to a vaidya, are unmistakable. Among the most obvious of these symptoms are dryness, stiffness, and bloating. More specifically, kapha imbalance robs the skin of moisture, leaving it dull and dry. The joints fall short of lubricant and become stiff. The tongue is coated with ama and the breath smells stale. The eyes look dull and devoid of ojas.

Another way in which a stressed body creates imbalance is by disturbing the vyana vata, the vata deputy that governs circulation, blood pressure, and the sense of touch. If your blood pressure is high, your nerves on edge, or your circulation sluggish, it is probably your vyana vata calling out for relief.

These distress signals can seem terribly alarming, but if you give your body some tender loving care the damage can be rapidly reversed. Start by making a list of the small ways in which you have been misusing or abusing your body. Are you giving it too much exercise, too little exercise, or not enough rest? Have you been reading in low light, watching television too closely, not sitting erect? If you answer "yes" to some or all of these questions, don't feel sorry. Instead, rejoice. You have done something remarkable: you have discovered the root cause of your stress. Now you can restore balance to your body without reaching for a pill or making a doctor's appointment.

De-stress Your Body in Three Easy Steps

1. Drink plenty of water. Nothing tones up the digestive system like a regular sip of lukewarm water. This is important because, more often than not, the stresses that burden the mind originate in the gut. Warm water helps flush out the toxins that throw kapha out of balance and lead to problems like bloating and water retention. At the same time, water balances vata, which, when aggravated, can cause stressful digestive problems like constipation. Water (at room temperature) also calms pitta, which, though blessed with a strong digestive fire, can be plagued by acidity and ulcers. The answer to all three problems: irrigate your body. Drink more water.

2. Take a fresh look at your daily quota of exercise. If you spend most of the day sitting at a desk, your digestion can slow down, encouraging toxins to build up inside your system. Therefore, you will benefit by working a moderate amount of exercise — an easy-paced twenty-minute walk, for example — into your schedule. On the other hand, too much exercise also throws the doshas out of balance. In that case, you should stop exerting and start making time for some rest.

3. Eat a peace-promoting snack. In Ayurveda, certain foods are identified as natural stress-busters. Among them are walnuts, almonds, coconut, lightly cooked juicy fruits like pears and apples, milk, fresh homemade yogurt, ghee, and fresh cheeses such as Indian-style homemade paneer (see recipe in chapter 9) or ricotta. If your body is feeling stressed, get more of these ingredients in your diet — based on a vaidya's assessment of which ones you need and how much.

move on to your mind

Do you think all the time but without clarity, work hard but without enthusiasm, and lie in bed without sleep? If yes, your stress has its origins in your mind. In Ayurvedic terms, these are classic symptoms of an out-of-balance vata — more specifically, the subdosha prana vata, or life force, that governs energy and calm.

When prana vata is disturbed, it impairs the mind's capacity to learn, retain, and recall information. Ayurveda has names for these three essential functions:

1. *dhi*, or acquisition of knowledge,
2. *dhriti*, or retention of knowledge, and
3. *smriti*, or recall of that knowledge.

Therefore, if you can register new information in a flash, make creative use of it in your work, and have a photographic memory; congratulate yourself. Your stress levels are wonderfully low and your mind's key coordinates are working in harmony.

But, given our overload of stresses, I doubt if many of us can afford to congratulate ourselves. I'm more familiar with the dhi/dhriti/smriti imbalance that shows up in little ways: going blank, forgetting our keys, struggling to remember a name. I know of someone who regularly forgets whether she has eaten her lunch!

Again, recovering from mental fatigue is not as frightening as it first looks. Philosopher and writer Franz Kafka, in fact, made it sound delightfully easy:

> You do not need to leave your room. Remain sitting at your table and listen. Do not even listen, simply wait. Do not even wait, be quite still and solitary. The world will freely offer itself to you to be unmasked, it has no choice, it will roll in ecstasy at your feet.

While such moments of quietude are no doubt divinely healing, they are hard to find. Take a more proactive approach: try the following simple ways to heal your unhappy prana vata.

Five Ways to Balance Your Prana Vata

1. Don't work long hours at the computer; it saps the mind of energy.
2. Don't stress over a niggling problem; it makes you lose your calm, thus disturbing prana vata.
3. Do get up and take a walk in between jobs; even a short break can restore calm in both body and mind.
4. Change coffee breaks into herbal-tea breaks. Good-quality Ayurvedic herbal teas (see resource list) contain healing herbs such as *brahmi, ashwagandha,* and *arjuna.* Extensive modern research has established that the herb brahmi enhances all three mental capacities: dhi, dhriti, and smriti. Ashwagandha is an effective weapon against physical fatigue. And arjuna heals the emotional aspect of the heart. Thus, just one cup of herbal tea can take you from stressed to rested within minutes.
5. Allow yourself the luxury of a nature walk, an evening spent among flowers, a healing nap. Such calming activities recharge your batteries and are very pleasing to prana vata.

examine your emotions

Do you notice a pattern so far? Physical stress is connected largely with a kapha imbalance, and mental stress with vata disturbance. Logically, then, emotional problems should be related to pitta, right? Right. More specifically, emotions are the terrain of the subdosha sadhaka pitta. But more about that in just a while.

Ayurveda recognizes that deep-seated stress is always related to emotional problems. The most common among them are marital conflicts or the loss of a loved one. Because the situation that creates emotional stress is generally traumatic, it is also more devastating than any other kind of stress. People going through emotional turmoil can suffer from chronic depression, highly toxic bottled-up anger, nightmares, and terrible insecurity. When that happens, it is time to pacify sadhaka pitta, the vital force that governs comfort, contentment, and emotional fulfillment.

Five Ways to Satisfy Your Sadhaka Pitta

1. Appease your sadhaka pitta with sweet, bitter, and astringent foods. (See chapter 7 to find a list of foods that fall in each of these categories.)
2. Comfort it with sweet, juicy fruits in the morning or during the day, delicately flavored sweet lassi in the afternoon, and warm milk at night.
3. Calm it with the healing goodness of cooling herbs and spices such as cardamom, cilantro, and mint.
4. Don't rush or skip lunch. To soothe between-meal

hunger pangs, snack on something wholesome like fruit or a whole-wheat bagel. Sadhaka pitta rules comfort, remember?

5. Turn down the noise in your life: switch off your mobile phone, take a day off work, give yourself permission to enjoy some moments of solitude.

Consult a vaidya for guidance if you feel that your stresses run too deep. Sometimes a vaidya will prescribe a nutritional supplement to awaken your body's immunity, strengthen your mind, and calm your emotions.

more stress solutions

In addition to these targeted remedies, Ayurveda has some excellent therapies that can vaporize any kind of stress — whatever its origin and intensity. Here are some key recommendations.

Get Good Sleep

When you deprive yourself of good sleep, you violate every law that is precious to Ayurveda: you cannot eat regular meals because your appetite is poor; this, in turn, slows down digestion, which results in toxin build-up; slowly, the toxins make you feel irritated and fatigued, and your strain affects your performance, your relationships, and your life. In such a state, you cannot hope to be creative, calm, or happy.

Ayurvedic healers studied sleep in great depth and

observed several natural rest-friendly aids. Here are some:

- Eat an early dinner. Avoid eating after 7:00 P.M., when digestion is slow and even light foods sit in the stomach and interfere with good sleep. Ideally, your physical digestive processes should be completed before you get into bed.

- Do some pre-sleep preparation. About an hour before you get into bed, start switching off heavy sensory inputs like the three-hankie tear-jerker on television. Such information accumulates ama in your mind, causing disturbed sleep. Now prepare for the night ahead: light some aromatic candles to create an ambiance of peace, listen to soft music, or just lie down and breathe deeply.

- Drink milk and honey. Just before you sleep, drink a glass of warm milk with a little honey in it. This has a settling influence on the mind and the body. Although this is an ancient remedy, modern medicine has now established the link between milk and good sleep: milk contains the amino acid tryptophan, which releases serotonin, a brain chemical that makes sleep come easily. Never heat honey, as this eliminates its beneficial qualities. Adding a pinch of nutmeg or cardamom to the milk also promotes better sleep.

- Go to bed early. Try to go to bed by 10:00 P.M.

If you are in the habit of staying up late, aim to achieve this in gradual stages: on the first night, try going to bed half an hour earlier than usual. This will help set your biomachinery in rhythm, promoting better rest. If you work night shifts, follow the rhythm of your body and mind, which will tell you when they need rest and how much. The simplest thing to do is: sleep when you feel sleepy.

- See a vaidya. If nothing works, consult a vaidya to help you determine what specific imbalance is disrupting your sleep.

Breathe Out Your Stresses

Have you ever noticed how you breathe when you are angry or depressed? Depending on the intensity of your mood, your breath at that time is shallow, rapid, or labored — never deep, calm, and relaxed. Again, this is a sign of imbalanced prana vata. It follows, therefore, that practicing the art of breathing properly will balance your vata and thus ease stress.

Ayurveda recommends some easy and effective breathing exercises — the most important among them being *pranayama* (regulation of life force). This is how you do it:

1. Sit straight and comfortably.
2. Now gently press your right nostril with your right thumb, shutting the nostril.
3. At the same time, breathe out slowly through

your left nostril until you have exhaled a full
breath.

4. Now breathe in through your left nostril and,
   once you have inhaled completely, release your
   right nostril and press the left one with the
   middle and ring fingers of the right hand.

5. Breathe out gently through the right nostril,
   then breathe slowly in again.

6. Repeat this rhythm for five minutes, and you
   will feel your body and mind become relaxed
   and healed.

Do this exercise whenever you can find five minutes,
and you will find it extremely soothing to your nerves.

Heal with Herbs

Herbs are a highly venerated tool in Ayurvedic healing. Rich in antioxidants, they are mighty fighters, capable
of calming the deadliest of stresses. Of course, Western
medicines are also largely herb-based. But the way
Ayurvedic herbal formulations are prepared is different
from the way they are prepared in modern laboratories.

To explain, let me ask you a question: Can a car move
without its wheels — or its gears, or the engine? In the
same way, an herb cannot heal without all its component
parts. This is where vaidyas say modern medicine errs.
Isolating and minutely studying a plant's "active" ingredients, it assigns them individual roles in treating disease.
While this "magic bullet" approach works, it also triggers a series of side effects, listed in curled-up slips of
paper inside medicine bottles.

The Ayurvedic disagreement with this method of treatment begins with the use of the word *active*. Vaidyas argue that there is no such thing as an *inactive* ingredient. Every ingredient in every plant has a definite role; even the seemingly inactive ones serve to balance the functions of the "active" ingredients. That is why, imbued with nature's own abundant intelligence, the plant kingdom has survived and thrived through the ravages of time.

Ayurveda's herbal formulas, therefore, enter the body as intended by nature herself. This is not to say they aren't processed; they are also ground into powders and pastes, but they are prepared in conformance with the stringent guidelines laid down in ancient texts. Therefore, good-quality Ayurvedic preparations retain their intrinsic synergy. When such preparations enter the human body, it greets them enthusiastically because it recognizes their configuration. Metabolizing and absorbing these holistic plant compounds is easy for the body because they carry their own balancing codes. That is why Ayurvedic medication is generally free of side effects.

A word of caution: Always take herbal preparations after consulting a vaidya. Never experiment with herbs on your own, for they can be quite potent if they are not balanced in the correct proportions with the right companion herbs.

Find Peace through Panchakarma

There are times when stress can take you to a breaking point. You feel saturated with demands, yet completely empty. Regard such times as the perfect opportunity to rebuild yourself the Ayurveda way.

In Ayurveda, it is understood that everyday toxins can build up to a point where they need removal through trained hands. In fact, regular seasonal rejuvenation is a unique and important Ayurvedic concept. It is called *panchakarma*, which literally means "five actions" (emesis, or vomiting, purgation, enemas, nasal cleansing, and blood purification). Today, however, panchakarma experts usually avoid inducing vomiting — the therapies they administer are pleasant, relaxing, and detoxifying. These include herbal massages and baths, light meals, steam baths, and herbal-paste rubs. All are designed to remove deep-seated toxins from your physiology, leaving you stress-free and renewed.

Ancient Ayurvedic texts recommend taking the panchakarma treatment three times a year, at the beginning of winter, spring, and fall. But if you find it expensive — and panchakarma can be heavy on the wallet — even once a year is highly beneficial and well worth the expense. Spring is said to be the best time for panchakarma treatment, for it is the season when everything in nature sheds its lethargy and starts to rejuvenate. The entire procedure takes about a week — and it leaves you so rejuvenated that you won't want to leave!

While panchakarma is an elaborate, complex therapy and thus best explained in detail by the physicians at a panchakarma center, I'll give you a basic idea of what to expect from it. You could think of the panchakarma routine either as a treatment or a treat. Either way, you would be right.

This is how panchakarma is generally done: You start on the road to rejuvenation a few days before you actually check into a panchakarma center. Ayurvedic experts interview you and outline for you a set of personalized instructions on how to start loosening impurities from your body. Easy to follow, these home-based therapies — such as drinking ghee, reducing your caloric intake, and using mild laxatives — are geared to prepare you for the wonderful detoxifying therapies you will receive in the panchakarma clinic.

Once in the clinic — where you can opt to be either an inpatient or an outpatient — you will receive a series of treatments designed to flush out long-accumulated toxins from your entire being.

The sequence begins with a full-body, warm-oil massage administered by two trained experts working in tandem. A good panchakarma center will generally use the highest-quality, cold-pressed, herb-infused oil for this part of the treatment. These special oils can sometimes contain up to seventy-five different herbs — which, when rubbed expertly into your body, stimulate skin cells, smooth away fat deposits, enliven the tissues, and — as Ayurveda's founder Charaka said — "give you 100 years of life."

Along with the oil massage, you will receive massages with whole-grain paste, raw silk, or wool, which further purify, tone, and nourish your body at a deep cellular level.

Then your nasal passages are cleared with drops of *nasya*, or medicated oil. These tiny drops unclog residual toxins from your head and neck, balancing the prana (essential energy or life force) that is so vital to clarity of perception.

The crowning glory in the panchakarma process, however, is *shirodhara* (*shir* means "head," and *dhara* means "flow"). Two therapists work in tandem, pouring a continuous stream of herbalized oil gently across your forehead. For thirty relaxing minutes, you do nothing but lie there with your eyes closed, feeling the stress slide right off your head. The oil used is blended with careful attention to the needs of your physiology. This treatment settles and balances the nervous system. Those who have experienced it describe it variously as "royal," "divine," and "utterly blissful." After shirodhara, you are likely to feel your anxiety, insomnia, and depression dissolve.

The massage therapies are followed by toxin-loosening heat-treatments such as *swedana*, which is an herbalized steam bath that dilates your shrotas, or channels of circulation. Swedana balances both vata and kapha doshas (pitta can do without additional heat), allowing the loosened impurities to move into the digestive tract in readiness for their removal by internal cleansing procedures.

By now, the impurities in your system have moved to the colon and lower pelvis, from where they will be further swept out through gentle herb-based enemas. Called *basti*, this part of the treatment is crucial to healing. The enemas used in basti are either made from warm herbalized oils or from water-based herbal decoctions — either way, they are very gentle and healing.

This then, is the promise of panchakarma. Some of its treatments calm the mind, while others cleanse and tone the body. Together they restore the functional integrity of your being. Your three doshas begin to work in harmony, and your endocrine system starts to perform at peak efficiency. Having flushed out its long-accumulated impurities, your immune system is stronger than ever. After panchakarma, you will exude ojas, or essential energy. Once you have taken a panchakarma treatment, experts advise daily detoxification at home through simple routines such as drinking plenty of water and giving yourself a daily pre-bath massage. This maintains, and even enhances, the benefits you receive from panchakarma.

Do you see how holistically Ayurveda heals stress — how perfectly it tunes the violin of your being, stretching the strings just right; not too loose, not too tight? Panchakarma makes it easy for you to close your eyes and enjoy the music that flows spontaneously in your being.

In the next chapter, we shall learn about yoga — another gem in Ayurveda's treasury of holistic healing therapies.

yoga: an exercise in bliss

Yogah chittah vritti nirodhah. (*Yoga is the ability to direct the mind exclusively, free of distractions.*)

— Patanjali's Yoga Sutra

What is yoga? The answers vary. According to Patanjali's Yoga Sutra:

- "It is a series of exercises that promotes neuro-muscular integration."
- "It is a system of healing that complements Ayurveda perfectly, having originated at the same time, in the same place, with the same goals."
- "It is a time-tested regimen that balances all three doshas, vata, pitta, and kapha."

More simply, yoga is a workout that has more than 15 million Americans hooked.

Of course, yoga stretches make great exercises; they're gentle, they're artistic, and they help you live better in your body. But more than that, I would say yoga works on the joints of the mind-body machine, lubricating them with the balm of consciousness.

The truth of this grandiose-sounding statement shines forth when you try the most primary of yoga poses. For instance, this one:

- Sit on the floor and cross your legs.
- Keep your spine straight.
- Now bring your palms to chest level and gently press them together, fingers pointing up.
- Close your eyes and breathe in, then breathe out. Breathe slowly in, breathe out again. Breathe in, breathe out.

At this moment, you are aware of your breathing. You are aware, too, of your body — your legs folded, your back straight, your palms pressed together. And you are conscious of the thoughts coursing through your mind.

This is what yoga does. It yokes your body, mind, and spirit together. In fact, the very origin of the word "yoga" is *yuj*, a Sanskrit word that means "to bind or unite." The English work *yoke*, which means to "tie together," is probably derived from this, too. Sage Patanjali, who codified the basic principles of yoga into his immortal Yoga Sutras, saw in yoga a deeper meaning. He saw it as a means to unite the Self with the Divine.

But can you really think of things like unity and harmony when trying to squeeze in a yoga class between a bath and a business meeting? No sweat. Yoga will reward you with harmony anyway — whether you search for it or not. My friend Bob Rose, a longtime yoga instructor, has had the pleasure of seeing hundreds of people discover deeper bliss in their lives through yoga. That experience of bliss can be so pure, so profound, that it often inspires poetic praise. For some people, yoga turns out to be "a joyful workout that untangles the mind." Others find in it "dynamic nirvana." And still others realize that it helps them "navigate the landscape of the self."

The truth is, yoga works because it works on every level of your being. Physically, it helps you touch your toes and sit straight. It unjumbles knotted-up joints, creating a sense of openness and fluidity in the body. It stimulates digestion and improves blood flow. It is a wonderful aid to any weight-loss program. It helps you breathe more consciously. In Ayurvedic terms, yoga is an excellent way to exercise because it does not put strain on any one part of the physiology. Besides, it heals and calms all three doshas.

On the mental level, yoga brings together two diametrically opposed energies: it makes you feel relaxed and easy of mind, and at the same time it teaches you discipline. It makes you more aware of your body, your thoughts, and emotions. It connects you with your very spirit.

What's more, yoga yields even richer rewards if you have some knowledge of its sister science: Ayurveda.

yoga and ayurveda – inseparably bound

As we saw, a vaidya's prescription is a holistic one. In addition to diet, it tells you to regulate your work routine, your quota of sleep, and your pattern of exercise. Yoga comes under that important heading of exercise.

Basically, the yoga exercises you choose to do should complement the diet and lifestyle recommendations that a vaidya charts out for you. If you are a vata type of person, for instance, backward bends are beneficial for you; they are believed to offset the coolness of vata. Pitta type of people will like postures that involve bending forward, for they cool down the system. And kapha will enjoy poses that involve twisting the body, for such poses kickstart digestion.

Five Ways in Which Ayurveda Supports Yoga

Along with matching your yoga exercises to your body type, you can also match them to your daily routine.

1. One of the primary benefits of yoga is that it starts to push toxic ama from your system. Now, while your body is flushing out toxins, your knowledge of Ayurveda can prove invaluable in assisting your body. It will guide you toward foods that are considered light and nourishing: split yellow lentils, sweet juicy fruits, plenty of water.

2. Using ghee in daily cooking, which is a basic Ayurvedic recommendation, supports yoga exercises. Ghee has been believed since ancient times to lubricate connective tissues and increase flexibility. So if you are learning yoga and cooking with ghee, you are getting the maximum benefits of both Ayurveda and yoga.

3. Daily self-massage, or abhyanga, is part of a healthy Ayurvedic routine (see chapter 10 for details). Among the many benefits of self-massage is that it moves toxins from the body, helping flush them out of your system through the channels of elimination. So if you massage your body regularly in conjunction with yoga exercises, you will give a much greater boost to toxin removal.

4. Ayurveda emphasizes the value of eating breakfast, lunch, and dinner at regular hours to keep toxins from building up. A person who knows this will take care to supplement her yoga sessions with healthy meals at scheduled mealtimes.

5. There are times when the body feels too sapped to exercise, even gently, or when the mind is too tired to focus on anything at all. These are times when Ayurvedic herbs prove to be of tremendous value. Powerful healers such as ashwagandha and arjuna have long been known to strengthen both body and mind. Blended in the right proportions and taken as recommended

by a vaidya, these herbs provide vital support to your yoga practice.

the practice of yoga

Yoga asanas are poses or exercises designed to work your body in a series of non-strenuous steps. The key in yoga exercises is to begin slowly, progress steadily toward the next step, and relax after every asana.

Almost every yoga asana contributes in its own way to making you more beautiful, because each of them helps strengthen several aspects of body and mind. I will share with you three favorites, which are not only easy but extremely relaxing.

sun salute (surya namaskar asana)

How to Do It: Sun Salute is performed in twelve continuous stages:

1. Standing up, with feet close together, place the palms and fingers of your hands together in front of your chest, fingers pointing upward. Breathe normally, looking forward, for five seconds.
2. Unclasp your hands and, inhaling slowly, raise them parallel to each other, shoulder-width apart, over your head with palms facing forward. Extend your arms slightly behind your head so that your waist is slightly bent and your face is tilted toward the ceiling or sky.

Hold your position, as well as your
breath, for another five seconds.

3. Exhaling, lean slowly forward and
touch the floor in front of your feet.
Do this only to the extent that you
can. Keep your hands about shoulder-
width apart and bring your head as
close to your knees as you can without
straining any muscles. Keep your knees
straight. Hold this position and your
exhaled breath for the next five seconds.

4. Inhale once again, and simultaneously
place your palms on the floor shoulder-width
apart. You'll find it easy to do this while sending your right leg straight
back, with its knee and
toes touching the floor.
Bring the left leg forward
at a ninety-degree angle to
the floor, so that your left knee is a little below
your chin. Arch your back and tilt your neck up
toward the ceiling or sky. Hold this position
and your breath for five seconds.

5. Now start exhaling while placing your left leg
back with the right leg. At the same time, raise
your buttocks and hips so they form a mound
shape, pointing straight
up. Your palms and fingers
should still be held flat on
the floor, and your head

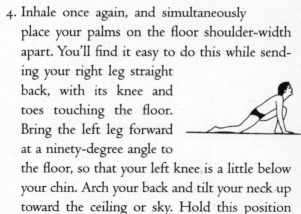

between your arms. Try to get your feet flat on the floor at this time — but try very gently. Remember, no strain. Again, hold your breath in this position for five seconds.

6. Slowly releasing your breath, lower your chin, chest, and knees until they almost touch the floor

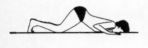

and the weight of your body is briefly on your palms and toes. Keep your hips raised above the floor. You don't have to maintain this position; make the transition to the next one once you have reached this one.

7. The next part is called the Cobra pose. Keep your palms in place. While inhaling,

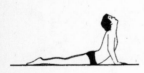

straighten your arms, arch your neck and spine so that your head tilts back, and keep your knees and toes touching the floor. Once you reach this position, hold your breath here for five seconds.

8. Repeat position 5: exhale while raising your hips and buttocks to point straight up. Keep your

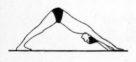

knees and back straight, palms on the floor, head between your arms. Hold for five seconds.

9. Return to position 4: keeping your hands on the floor, bend your left leg at the knee while inhaling. The right knee and toes should stretch

behind you, touching the
floor. Arch your back and
neck to gaze upward. Hold
another five seconds.

10. Step your back foot forward beside your other
    foot, returning to position 3: exhale,
    straighten your knees, bend forward
    at the waist and hips. Your full weight
    is now back on your feet. Try to touch
    the floor with your palms once again
    without undue effort. Keep your head
    close to your knees. Hold this posi-
    tion and your breath for five seconds.

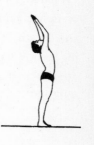

11. Repeat position 2: begin exhaling
    as you raise the upper half of your
    body until you are standing straight
    again. Raise your arms above your
    head with the palms facing forward.
    Continue to stretch your arms until
    they are slightly behind your head,
    then lean slightly back from the
    waist and gaze upward, holding your
    breath for five seconds.

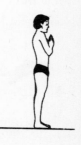

12. Go back to position 1, then slowly
    exhale (instead of inhaling). Stand
    straight, with palms and fingers
    held together in front of your chest
    and your eyes looking straight in
    front of you. Hold your breath out
    for five seconds.

Here are some additional tips on performing Sun Salute:

- When you do the second set of this asana, take the alternate leg back in positions 4 and 9. That is, in the sequence above, you extended your right leg backward; in the next set, take your left leg backward.
- Try to do this asana in even sets of two, four, or six, up to a maximum of twelve at a time.
- Always do this in a slow, steady manner without causing yourself strain. Build up your threshold gradually.

What It Does for You: Sun Salute, as you can see, is a complete asana that involves all parts of the body, mind, and breath. It thus integrates the physiology, strengthening major muscles and providing a light yet complete exercise that vaidyas recommend as highly as they do walking.

child's pose (balasana)

How to Do It: Kneel on your shins, buttocks resting on your heels. Keep your knees together. With your arms at

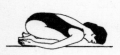

your sides, bend from your hips and extend your upper body over your knees. Resting on your thighs, bring your forehead to the floor. Breathe deeply. Hold for as long as is comfortable. Then slowly sit up.

If you have trouble kneeling, placing a pillow between your thighs and calves will help.

What It Does for You: This simple asana floods every cell of the body with both oxygen and prana (life-force energy), helping eliminate physical and emotional toxins. The constriction on your legs increases blood supply to the upper body, making respiration more efficient and energizing the blood, which in turn begins to remove waste gases more efficiently. The pressure from the diaphragm in this posture creates a deep, slow, rhythmic massage of the vital organs, energizing them. Both the quality and quantity of the blood circulation to these vital organs improves when you are in Child's Pose.

If you hold the pose for more than five minutes, deeper benefits occur. The asana has a regulatory effect on the endocrine system. It gets more blood to the head and to the pituitary gland — the master gland that regulates hormonal balance. This makes Child's Pose an extremely relaxing asana.

corpse pose (shavasana)

It sounds like the easiest thing you could do: lying there like your body is dead to the world. But yoga experts tell me that this is among the most difficult asanas to master because we humans find it so difficult to allow ourselves to just let go and lie still.

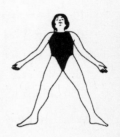

Before he starts his instructions for the asana itself, yoga instructor Bob Rose tells his students to put all their anger, anxieties, and tensions in an imaginary bag that they mentally place outside the door. The choice is theirs, he tells them — you can leave the bag there when you go out, or pick it back up if you desire.

How to Do It: Lie on your back, with your feet about eighteen inches apart and turned out slightly. Place your hands on the floor about six inches from your hips, palms up. Close your eyes and breathe deeply and gently.

Rose likes to tell his students to do this asana in three "let-go" phases:

1. Let go of your body: Relax your muscles and any tense areas by breathing deeply and gently and directing your breath to those tense areas. Let your muscles sink right into the floor until they're so relaxed they feel like Jell-O.

2. Let go of your breathing: After you have used your breath to relax your body, then let the breathing process become as gentle and natural as possible. Don't control it. Relax, yawn, sigh. Let it become as deep or shallow as it wants to be.

3. Let go of your thoughts: Release yourself from thinking. This does not mean making an effort to banish them. Just let yourself become a passive observer — watching your thoughts go by like clouds in the sky.

What It Does for You: This asana is a luxury we don't allow ourselves — a few minutes of just being, not doing. The very act of consciously relaxing — lying still, fully present in the moment — begins the process of releasing knots of tension from the deep recesses of the body and mind. It's more than an asana; it's a form of meditation, which slows down the metabolism, lowers blood pressure, and leaves you with a feeling of deep calm and rest.

some general tips on practicing yoga

- Always relax for a minute or two after every asana.
- Do not practice yoga on a full stomach or just before a meal.
- Ideally, perform yoga in the morning, right after a bath.
- Do yoga without listening to music or watching television. Yoga is a wonderful way to focus on your body and its various components, so you will benefit more from it if you do it without distraction.
- If you are menstruating, pregnant, ill, or have some specific bodily disorders, see a qualified yoga practitioner for guidance.
- For best results, perform yoga exercises daily.

yoga: frequently asked questions

When and How Did Yoga Originate?

Yoga has always been an integral part of the Indian civilization. The world's oldest existing text, Rig-Veda, mentions it. But the credit for defining and organizing yoga is widely given to Sage Patanjali, who lived sometime around 200 A.D. In his treatise, called the Yoga Sutras, Patanjali lays down the philosophy, goals, and rules of yoga.

What Are the Different Kinds of Yoga, and Which One Is for Me?

The most popular form of yoga today is hatha yoga. The word *hatha* means "insistence." In the context of hatha yoga, the meaning of insistence is slightly modified; it means making consistent effort toward healing the self through simple postures and exercises. The exercises taught in hatha yoga are called asanas, some of which I have described above.

Other branches of yoga include raja yoga, karma yoga, bhakti yoga, jnana yoga, tantra yoga, and mantra yoga. These are all more evolved forms of yoga that delve into the realm of the spiritual. Most of the yoga classes in America are for hatha yoga.

Where Can I Learn More about Yoga?

I would recommend the magazine *Yoga Journal*, which combines articles on Ayurveda with fine writing on every aspect of yoga. In addition, introductory texts such as the *K.I.S.S Guide to Yoga* (DK publishing) are also very helpful. Another comprehensive book that discusses the mind-body benefits of yoga and its connection with Ayurveda is Hari Sharma's *Contemporary Ayurveda* (Churchill Livingstone).

living ayurveda, giving ayurveda

Every person in your life, all the events,
are there because you have drawn them there.
What you choose to do with them is up to you.

— Richard Bach, *Illusions*

Have you noticed something about the Ayurvedic approach to life thus far? It seems to have a great fondness for clichés — timeworn statements that seem to us so hackneyed that we don't even think about them. "A stitch in time saves nine." "Early to bed and early to rise." "You are what you eat." And so on.

Hackneyed, yes. But outdated, no. Each little nugget of Ayurvedic wisdom, you will agree, is timeless — and hence, invaluable. From my own experience of Ayurveda, I've spun seven sparkling, er, clichés.

living ayurveda

1. Eat Fresh, Eat Red, Yellow, Green

We've talked about this before, but let me leave you with yet another reason to rethink your grocery shopping list. Look at the peach. It is a painter's delight. Why do you think nature made it so attractive? Those crimson apples, flaming peppers, young green spinach leaves — ever wondered if all that color scheming has a purpose? Well, it certainly does. By putting those colors on its plants, nature is beckoning you to notice them, yield to their lure, savor them. Perhaps that is one of the reasons why humans are the only creatures gifted with color vision; almost all other animals see in black-and-white.

Take time today to think about the food choices you make. The entire technology of the food industry is only trying to imitate the oldest marketing technique on earth. All that creative energy and, of course, billions of dollars are being spent on designing attractive, colorful labels for stripped-down, almost-dead food — while living, pulsating food screams silently for attention. Why strip and repackage the brilliant original? Bite into a luscious peach today.

2. Stay Fit, Stay Lean

Ayurveda does not advocate toning up just the abs or focusing on the pectoral muscles. Truly fit people are trim and toned all over. Work toward fitness without flogging your body. Remember, walking and yoga are considered the most healing exercises in Ayurveda.

As for staying lean, cancel your weight-management-program membership and let your own mind be your coach. The reason for weight gain is simple: you are eating more than you are burning up. To keep your calorie intake balanced, just remember the rule of three-fourths: fill your stomach to three-fourths of its capacity at any one meal, and you will never be in danger of overeating. Basically, eat to feel satisfied, not to feel full and heavy.

A word about ghee. Ayurvedic experts do recommend cooking with ghee, but they caution that generous dollops of ghee can clog the system, increase kapha, and pile on the pounds. Used in moderation, on the other hand, ghee will endow you with health benefits.

3. Live Life Clean

Being clean in body means observing good personal hygiene. Bathe every day. Wear fresh clothing. Always respond to a natural urge: hunger, thirst, or the need to yawn, sneeze, or urinate. These are natural instincts that deserve prompt attention. Suppressing them, according to Ayurveda, generates toxins and stresses the body.

Keep your mind clean: read uplifting books, watch movies that leave you with a smile in your heart, delete junk mail, and listen to music, not noise.

Keep your heart clean: don't envy others their success; keep an even temper; don't play the blame-game; be open to sunshine and love.

4. Adopt the Golden Mean

Ayurveda is essentially about balance. The Golden Mean is "the medium between extremes," or "moderation."

And in the thesaurus, "balance" and "moderation" are neighbors.

Long ago, I had a poster in my room. It said: "If it feels good, overdo it." I loved that poster. I took it so seriously that I overloaded on guavas that someone had given us. They tasted so delicious that I ate ten at one sitting. The stomachache that followed was not fun. This is a simplistic example, but the Ayurvedic insistence on "moderation in everything" is a golden rule, indeed. Quite simply, people who eat, sleep, work, think, and love either too much or too little are not healthy, happy people.

5. Keep Your Appetite Keen

Rev up your appetite. Fix up your dining room. Make a trip to your local library and borrow some good books and magazines on the art of decoration. Then turn the spotlight on the most appetizing corner of your home: your dining table.

Bring out your best china and your most exclusive cutlery. Light some scented, all-natural candles. Place a vase of fresh flowers or a bowl of fresh fruit in the center of the table. Accent with colorful napkins and place mats. Now invite a friend over to share a simple, home-made meal.

This might sound like advice from the pages of *House & Garden*. But it has a beautiful Ayurvedic message, too: creating a beautiful dining environment makes the act of eating a pleasurable, sacred one.

Eat foods that you enjoy. That we're talking about healthy foods is, of course, a given. If your taste buds like what you eat, your body will digest it more efficiently. In India, we say *aisa khana badan ko lagta hai* — "such food is infused into the body much more completely."

Now apply this keenness of appetite to wider areas of your life. Get hungry for knowledge. Read up on health. Learn about the world. Travel. Open your mind and your heart to the splendor of the universe. One cliché Ayurveda does not promote is: "Ignorance is bliss"!

6. Seek the Serene

Peace, calm, positive energy — these are found in people who have qualities of the sattva guna. Even in the animal kingdom, there are species that represent the three gunas — rajas, tamas, and sattva. Ayurvedic healers use the imagery of the tiger, the jackal, and the elephant to illustrate the value of sattva.

- The tiger represents the rajasic nature. He is a carnivore, and this natural instinct of killing and eating other animals makes him fierce and aggressive. Powerful and restless, the tiger is always on the prowl, always looking for action.
- The jackal symbolizes the tamasic mind. He is sly, timid, and slothful, evading the clear light of day and preying on food left over by other animals.
- The elephant harbors a gentle heart inside a strong body. He is intelligent enough to work in harmony with the human environment. He is also a vegetarian. Therefore, the elephant represents the sattvic mind.

Notice how the diets of these animals are also linked to their mental qualities. Consider these qualities before selecting your next meal or deciding on your next course of action.

7. Don't View Life through a Smoke Screen

Can you imagine touring a lush national forest without ever stepping out of your car — leaving for home without ever touching the bark of the sequoia tree, photographing a moose, or smelling the pure, clean air? Most of us would laugh at the very idea. But aren't we doing the same thing with our lives? We're so busy chugging along the rails that lead to money, success, and love that we forget the pleasures of living life barefoot, so to speak.

On one hand, we set ourselves ephemeral goals. On the other, we dull our senses with information overload. I recently found a rather staggering statistic in a health magazine. It said that an average American watches television for about 240 minutes a day. Four hours of watching other people act, inform, sell, emote — in a mere twenty-four-hour day? It's ironic when you think that the number-one excuse people give for neglecting their health is, well, "lack of time"!

Switch off the TV and tune in to yourself. If you are hopelessly hooked, cut down on your TV-watching time gradually — say, by fifteen minutes a day. In these fifteen minutes, treat yourself to a tall glass of water, some light stretching exercises, or just the healing sounds of silence. In Ayurvedic terms, this will reduce misuse of your senses, allowing your body to overcome stress.

Thus, truly rested, you can think more clearly about your life and its real purpose.

These seven guidelines sum up most of what Ayurveda has to say about good living. If you're able to follow even a few, you'll find your life improving in many ways.

---

the power of one

Let me share with you an interesting health strategy I have chalked out for myself. I call it The Power of One.

On days when I feel I've been neglecting almost every aspect of my health, I find a minute to sit down and write myself three resolutions. These are not resolutions for the rest of the year or even the rest of the month or week. They're goals I set for myself for the next thirty minutes. For instance:

1. Drink two glasses of water.
2. Exercise for five minutes.
3. Do someone a favor.

Now, life being what it is, it is not always possible to achieve even these seemingly simple targets. Once I realized this, I told myself I'd be happy if I could do even one of those three things; in however small a way, I would only be helping myself.

It works — first, because it's truly easy. And also because even the smallest positive action toward self-improvement makes you feel really, really good. That in itself adds a pinch of sattva to your being. Often, you'll find that if you're feeling good about yourself, you won't even have to remind yourself to help someone else; you'll just spontaneously do it.

---

giving ayurveda: seven aah-inspiring gift ideas

---

*It's not how much we give,
but how much love we put into giving.*

— Mother Teresa

Before I discovered Ayurveda, I seldom thought beyond picture frames, flowers, and cut-glass vases as gifts for my friends and family. Over the years, however, I have realized that there is no greater joy than giving the gift of well-being. Birthday or wedding anniversary, holiday season or for simply no reason — I always, always pick up something that I know will make my friends and family a little healthier. Bonus: the gift and its goodness evoke in people a curiosity about Ayurveda — and knowing what a world of difference Ayurveda can make, I am always happy to share what I know.

The Personal Touch

Some of the most beautiful moments in life come just after you have given someone a thoughtful gift. The sight of a parent's or friend's eyes lighting up, the spontaneous smile that spreads across their face — the pleasure it brings makes gift-giving something of a selfish act, too!

Along with your gift, include a handwritten note about its goodness. You could jot down quotations, make up your own poems (I made up this one: "Stop that nerve going bang-bang — soothe it down with ylang-ylang!"), or type some Ayurvedic advice in an old-style font, then print it out and paste it on the package.

Happily, there are scores of heartwarming Ayurvedic gifts you can think of. Let me share some favorite ones with you. Here's hoping these ideas will change the way you give — for the better, forever.

Something Scent-imental

I used to refrain from presenting perfume to people, thinking the gift would be forgotten once the scent had evaporated. But now I know that scent is something that stays with us; it can be an everlasting gift. And there is a perfectly scientific explanation for that.

Where does a smell go once it has stolen up the nostrils? It travels to the hypothalamus, and to some key areas of the brain that surround it — areas that process feelings and memories. That is why the fragrance of a rose lifts the spirits, and the scent of earth just after rain can remind you of happy long-ago times.

In the Ayurvedic world of healing, too, scents have a special place. Sweet orange, fennel, and ylang-ylang have a calming influence; they pacify the vata dosha. Rose, sandalwood, and lavender bring feelings of cool restfulness, which makes them perfect for pleasing a pitta person. And an unhappy kapha loves to be comforted by eucalyptus, rosemary, and basil.

Then there are herbs that can ease away muscle tension and soothe aching joints. Among the most effective are nutmeg, basil, spearmint, camphor, pine, and peppermint. That is why healing with natural aroma is an integral part of Ayurveda.

Give a Gift of Serenity

Pick and pack a favorite essential oil, an aroma diffuser, or an herbal neck-wrap. Stitch a cheerful cushion and fill it with healing, fragrant herbs. A tip for making your gift of oils extra special: read some good books on the healing properties of different oils, then try blending them for maximum benefit (see resources for some recommendations). Blended in the right proportions, essential oils yield synergistic benefits and balance each other out. Attach a note about how you discovered that ylang-ylang complements rose, or why rosemary and lavender make perfect companions. Thus prepared, your gift will give a lot of pleasure — not only to your friends, but also to you. Ah, the alchemy of aroma!

Bottled Bliss

Pure, organic, cold-pressed sesame oil makes a thoughtful gift — particularly for those who can obviously use some lubrication on their skin. Observe the skin texture of your family and friends. Parched, thirsty skin will love being treated to a deep moisturizing massage.

Then there's another kind of massage that needs no oil. Dry massage is a great way to exfoliate skin and boost sluggish circulation. Done regularly, this energizing massage can reduce the cottage-cheese appearance of cellulite. How about giving your friend a pair of raw silk gloves for performing a dry self-massage?

A Jugful of Joy

There are things in life that one doesn't usually think about. Your glass of water, for instance. You notice the water, but the glass itself is just a container. Some years ago, when I was staying with an aunt back in India, I noticed that she observed a nightly ritual. She would fill a copper jug with water and leave it overnight. Then, in the morning, she would pour herself two glasses of water from that jug. I thought she loved her copper jug simply because it was so pretty. Then she told me that leaving the water overnight in that jug enriched the fluid with the goodness of copper. It helped reduce acidity, improve digestion, and enhance the body's ability to assimilate food better.

So distribute health by the glassful: give your friends a copper cup.

A Basket of Apples

Your friend has been missing breakfast. She often looks tired and distracted. Or maybe she has just been working too hard these past few days to pay attention to her health. Put her back on the path to radiance: give her some apples or pears. Buy fresh, organic, sweet fruit. Make a bundle of cloves, and jot down the recipe for stewed apple/pear (see chapter 9, where you'll also find information on how a stewed fruit makes the perfect start for a day).

A Sachet of Spice

If your friend's idea of a spice box is the salt and pepper shakers, introduce her to the wonder of Ayur-vedic spices. To begin with, introduce her to the queen of spices: turmeric. In its solid form, turmeric looks like twisted yellow sticks. In India, many housewives like to grind it fresh each time they use it. But you could also buy good-quality turmeric in an Asian grocery store. Attach a recipe for cooking with turmeric, adding infor-mation on how it helps boost the immune system, flush out toxins, and aid digestion.

If your friend finds her new-look yellow veggies and curries appetizing, gradually introduce her to other stars in the Indian spice box: cumin, coriander, cardamom, and more.

A Gift of Sereni-tea!

Ayurvedic practice includes avoiding such caf-feinated drinks as coffee and tea. They are thought to overstimulate the mind and, taken in excess, disturb the balance of the doshas. Herbal teas, on the other hand, pack both flavor and healing qualities. The sweetness of licorice calms vata and pitta. Teas containing rose petals cool the pitta dosha, and those with cloves perk up a lethargic kapha. In general, Ayurvedic herbal teas zap fatigue, relax the mind, and calm the senses. Tea flavors like mint, lemon balm, and jasmine are so delectable that your friends can also try using them to flavor sauces and fruit-based desserts. You should be able to find some good herbal tea brands in natural food stores. Maharishi Ayurveda also makes some gourmet mind-body beverages for balancing each dosha type. (See resources for buying information.)

For the Thought Gourmet

To me, one of the most precious gifts is the gift of beautiful words: a collection of love poems, recipes, or short stories; a book of quotations; a life-changing novel; an inspiring book on natural healing. Choose from among some truly sensitive works that you have read and loved, books written with a sincerity that awakens the body's natural intelligence, stimulates the mind, and soothes the spirit. Giving away good health need not cost you a fortune. You could create a handmade booklet that is filled with health tips, recipe ideas, and beautiful pictures cut from old magazines.

I wish you a fulfilling lifetime of living and giving the priceless gift of Ayurveda!

surfing the ayurvedic ocean

*Each today, well-lived, makes yesterday a happy dream
and tomorrow a vision of hope.
Look, therefore, to this one day, for it and it alone is life.*

— Sanskrit poem

Before typing the first word of this book, I wanted to know what a reader would want from it. So I asked some friends to list their expectations. This was a diverse group of people; some had never heard of Ayurveda, others knew the definition but not much more, and still others had dipped their toes into the Ayurvedic waters but had hastily withdrawn them when they encountered the Sanskrit terminology. Here's a sampling of what they said:

- "I'd like to see a book that doesn't use any of those confusing terms."
- "I want to know whether Ayurveda can help me live a healthier life — and if yes, how. In plain English, please."
- "I cannot tell Ayurveda from chelation therapy, acupressure, and yoga. Please enlighten."

And so on.

I hope I have been able to write this book to the satisfaction of most of my friends. For those, however, who still feel that Ayurvedic terminology gets in the way of making it easily approachable, I have this to say: I understand your wariness completely.

For me, the journey toward Ayurveda posed fewer obstacles, for I had some basic advantages. Ayurveda and I were born in the same country. Hindi, a language derived from Sanskrit, is my mother tongue. My parents — and, more than them, my grandparents — understood Ayurveda by instinct.

Hence, I grew up hearing the proverbial wisdom of the Indian village. Some of those proverbs were gems in rhyme — so succinct and so wise that they're written in my mind with indelible ink. For example, my grandfather used to say, "A person who has a bowel movement once a day is a *yogi* [ascetic]. One who has it twice a day is a *bhogi* [taker of life's pleasures]. And one who has it thrice a day is a *rogi* [sick person]."

My grandmother would not let us eat cucumber salad in the evening, reciting this haiku-like poem:

Kheera
Subah ko heera
Din mein kheera
Raat mein peera.

It means, "A cucumber eaten in the morning has the goodness of a diamond, in the afternoon it has the benefits of cucumber, and in the evening, it is a source of pain."

Lunch was always given the highest priority. Come noon, my mother would want us to abandon anything we were doing — be it a math problem or a game — saying, *Pehle pet pooja, phir kaam dooja* ("first worship your stomach, then attend to other things").

I don't know how long ago these sayings were actually coined, or whether they came from Ayurvedic tradition at all. Whatever their origin, they later helped me understand Ayurveda and its aphorisms without feeling too surprised or skeptical. "Rise early." "Scrape your tongue." "Don't read while eating." These admonitions had always been part of my life; they were locked in my DNA, so to speak.

Even so, when I studied Ayurveda more formally it was somewhat of a daunting prospect. There were things that intimidated me about this system of healing:

- Its age. Ayurveda is, at the very least, more than 5,000 years old (some say it is a 10,000-year-old tradition, others say there's no way of knowing how old it really is). But even 5,000 years is a significant period of time, considering that we can barely visualize life as it must have been as recently as one hundred years ago.

- Its scale. Ayurvedic knowledge comes to us from comprehensive texts called *samhitas* and *nighantus*. Each one is an ocean in itself, and ancient Ayurvedic sages were prolific writers. Sage Atreya alone wrote 46,500 verses, all in Sanskrit — a language so scholarly that it is hard even for an Indian to learn.
- Its terminology. Doshas, dhatus, gunas — would I be able to wade through the vocabulary?
- Its complexity. Ayurvedic healers seemed to have had dozens of guidelines on every little thing. Drinking water, for instance: don't drink ice-cold water; don't drink warm water, either, if you're a pitta type; spice your water with cumin if you're a kapha type, and fennel if you're a vata; and so on.

But I am happy to say that my doubts and fears dissolved steadily. The more I studied Ayurveda, the more it resonated with my childhood years. Soon, I came to a delightful conclusion: Ayurvedic wisdom, in its purest essence, was a distilled version of my grandparents' admonitions.

From that epiphanic moment on, I was able to see Ayurveda as the majority of Indian people see it. In India, most people don't study Ayurveda. They live it in simple ways. When a child has a cold, her mother will steep some holy basil leaves in boiled water and have the child sip it at regular intervals. A sore throat is soothed with crushed black pepper stirred into honey. Food is cooked fresh, lavished with spices and herbs, then eaten hot. Because a daily bath is cleansing and healthy, many people accord it the status of a religious ritual — they will say their prayers and eat their first morsel of the day only after a bath. In these small ways, they live Ayurveda.

Even massage is an integral part of life in India; barbers-cum-masseurs are a common sight. Identifiable by the tool kit they carry, these barber/masseurs can be hailed on the streets. All they have to do is find a shady tree in the vicinity, and lo! A folding chair is pulled out, the kit is opened, and, a neat shave later, a relaxing head massage called *champi* is under way. At the other end of the spectrum are expensive herbal massage parlors, whose popularity is rising by the minute.

I hope that this book has helped you recognize that you can live Ayurveda, too.

In my own life, Ayurveda is a major influence; but I admit that my routine is often less than exemplary. There are times when I misuse my body — by going to bed late, watching TV too long, or slumping in my chair. When I'm rushed, I grab a muffin instead of stewed fruit. And I'm not above temper tantrums and arguments. But then, I don't allow these slipups to make me feel unduly guilty, because I know that Ayurveda does not mean constantly judging or berating oneself.

On the plus side, studying Ayurveda has made me give up carbonated sodas, canned beans, and bleached flour. I haven't tasted leftover food for many years now. I try not to bear a grudge. I'm learning to give people their space. And I have certainly grown more intuitive about my own body/mind needs.

Yet being a devotee of Ayurveda hasn't meant that I never see an allopathic doctor. In fact, Ayurveda works wonderfully with Western medicine as a complementary — or, more accurately — an integrative system of healing. If a vaidya thinks that your blood pressure is dangerously high or that you have a suspicious lump, you will probably be encouraged to see an allopathic doctor. And if a Western physician combines knowledge of modern medicine with the timeless wisdom of Ayurveda, the result can be an ideal healer. Happily, several Western physicians are doing this today.

That said, one thing is for sure: if you live Ayurveda in your daily life, you might not need to see a doctor — any doctor — at all, or at least not often.

I said in the beginning of this book that, to me, Ayurveda is an ocean — not just because it is so deep and vast, but also because it gives so many different things to different people. Ships sail across its bosom. Divers plunge in to look for treasures. Tourists stroll its beaches and heal themselves with its mist, its brilliant sunsets, its stillness.

Take from the Ayurvedic ocean what you can. Even its tiniest pearls will make you richer.

Let me leave you with a blessing that was meant quite literally in ancient India, because Ayurvedic sages believed that we humans were programmed to live at least a century:

Shatayu bhavah! (May you live a hundred years!)

dosha-wise food guide

These are basic guidelines only and are not intended to cover all possible food choices.

vata

General Guidelines

- You are slim and light in build, so you can afford to eat in good quantities. Just make sure you don't eat more than you can digest with ease.
- If you are trying to appease your vata, very few dairy products are off limits for you. So include butter, cheese, and milk in your diet.

- Unlike Kapha, which should avoid sweeteners, wiry vatas do well to get some sweeteners in their diet. But remember, moderation is the key.
- If your vata is strong, you already have plenty of dryness in your system. You need moist, sweet, luscious fruits, so eat dried fruits very sparingly. Avoid too much sun.
- Sweet, moist vegetables are excellent for balancing vata. In their raw form, they won't do you much good, so eat them cooked. Avoid gas-causing beans and vegetables such as broccoli and cauliflower in large quantities, for bloating and gas are associated with the "air" quality of vata.
- Most spices and nuts will do you good. For those you need to avoid, consult the list below.
- Balance the dryness of vata by using good-quality oils, both externally and in your cooking. Almost every oil works for this dosha.

fruits	
Friendliest	**Avoid**
Apples (cooked)	Apples (raw)
Applesauce	Cranberries
Apricots	Dates (dried)
Avocados	Figs (dried)
Bananas	Olives (green)
Berries	Pears
Cherries	Pomegranates
Coconut	Prunes (dried)
Dates (fresh)	Raisins (dried)
Figs (fresh)	Watermelon
Grapefruit	
Grapes	
Kiwi	
Lemons	
Limes	
Mangoes	
Melons	
Olives (black)	
Oranges	
Papaya	
Peaches	
Pineapple	
Plums	
Prunes (soaked)	
Raisins (soaked)	
Rhubarb	
Strawberries	
Tamarind	

vegetables			
Friendliest	Eat in Moderation	Okay if Eaten Rarely	Avoid
Asparagus	Cauliflower	Beet greens	Artichoke
Beets	(cooked)	Corn	Bitter melon
Cabbage	Daikon	Horseradish	Broccoli
(cooked)	radish	Tomatoes	Brussels sprouts
Carrots	(cooked)	(cooked)	Cabbage (raw)
Cilantro	Jerusalem		Cauliflower
Cucumber	artichoke		(raw)
Fennel	Leafy greens		Celery
Garlic	Lettuce		Eggplant
Green beans	Mustard		Kale
Okra	greens		Kohlrabi
Parsnips	Onions		Onions (raw)
Peas	(cooked)		Peppers (sweet
(cooked)	Parsley		and hot)
Pumpkin	Spinach		Potatoes
Rutabaga			(white)
Sweet			Prickly pear
potatoes			(fruit and
			leaves)
			Radishes (raw)
			Turnips
			Wheat-grass
			sprouts

legumes		
Friendliest	Eat in Moderation	Avoid
Mung beans (whole bean) Mung dal (split mung bean) Tur dal (split yellow lentils) Urad dal (split black lentils)	Lentils (red) Soy milk Soy sauce Tofu	Adzuki beans Black beans Black-eyed peas Chickpeas (garbanzo beans) Kidney beans Lentils (brown) Lima beans Navy beans Peas (dried) Pinto beans Soybeans Soy flour Soy powder Split peas Tempeh White beans

dairy products		
Friendliest	**Eat in Moderation**	**Avoid**
Butter	Cheese (hard)	Cow's milk
Buttermilk	Ice cream	(powdered)
Cheese (soft)	Sour cream	Goat's milk
Cottage cheese	Yogurt (diluted	(powdered)
Cow's milk	and spiced)	Yogurt (plain,
Ghee		frozen, or with
Goat cheese		fruit)
Goat's milk		

grains			
Friendliest	Eat in Moderation	Okay if Eaten Rarely	Avoid
Durum wheat flour Oats (cooked) Pancakes Quinoa Rice (all kinds) Wheat	Amaranth	Pasta Polenta Rice cakes	Barley Bread (with yeast) Buckwheat Cereal (cold, dry, or puffed) Corn Couscous Crackers Granola Millet Muesli Oat bran Oats (dry) Rye Sago Spelt Tapioca Wheat bran

beverages			
Friendliest	Drink in Moderation	Okay if Drunk Rarely	Avoid
Almond milk	Soy milk	Basil tea	Apple juice
Aloe vera	(hot and	Cinnamon	Black tea
juice	well-spiced)	tea	Caffeinated
Apple cider		Jasmine tea	beverages
Apricot juice		Lemon balm	Carbonated
Berry juice		tea	drinks
(except for		Prune juice	Chocolate milk
cranberry)		Tomato juice	Coffee
Carrot juice			Cold dairy
Chai (hot			drinks
spiced milk)			Cranberry juice
Chamomile			Ginseng tea
tea			Hibiscus tea
Cherry juice			Iced tea
Clove tea			Icy cold drinks
Grain "coffee"			Mixed vegetable
Grape juice			juice
Grapefruit			Pear juice
juice			Pomegranate
Lemonade			juice
Mango juice			Soy milk (cold)
Orange juice			Vegetable
Papaya juice			bouillon
Peach nectar			
Pineapple			
juice			
Rice milk			
Sour juices			

nuts	
Friendliest, but Best in Moderation	**Avoid**
Almonds Black walnuts Brazil nuts Cashews Hazelnuts Macadamia nuts Pecans Pine nuts Pistachios Walnuts	None

seeds	
Friendliest	**Avoid**
Flax Pumpkin Sesame Sunflower	Popcorn

spices, herbs, and condiments			
Friendliest		Okay in Moderation	Avoid
Ajwain	Mango pickle	Black pepper	Caraway
Allspice	Marjoram	Cayenne	Chocolate
Almond	Mint	Chili peppers	Horseradish
extract	Mustard	(dried)	
Anise	Mustard	Cilantro	
Asafetida	seeds	Fenugreek	
Basil	Nutmeg		
Bay leaf	Orange peel		
Black pepper	Oregano		
Cardamom	Paprika		
Chutney,	Parsley		
mango	Peppermint		
(sweet or	Poppy seeds		
spicy)	Rosemary		
Cinnamon	Saffron		
Cloves	Salt		
Coriander	Savory		
Cumin	Scallions		
Curry leaves	Seaweed		
Dill	Soy sauce		
Fennel	Spearmint		
Ginger	Star anise		
Ketchup	Tarragon		
Lemon	Thyme		
Lime	Turmeric		
Lime pickle	Vanilla		
Mace	Wintergreen		

oils		
Friendliest	External Use Only	Avoid
Ghee Olive Sesame Most other oils	Coconut Avocado	Flaxseed

sweeteners		
Friendliest	Okay if Used Rarely	Avoid
Barley malt Fructose Fruit-juice concentrate Honey (raw and not processed) Jaggery Molasses Rice syrup Turbinado	Maple syrup	White sugar

pitta

General Guidelines

- Balance an aggravated pitta with sweet dairy products such as milk, butter, and ghee. Avoid such sour dairy products as yogurt, cheese, sour cream, and buttermilk.

- You are a fiery dosha, so sweeteners of almost all kinds are great for balancing you out. Go slow on honey and molasses, though.

- Counter the heat of pitta with sweet, ripe, juicy fruits. Stay away from sour fruits. Similarly, avoid vegetables that are hot (peppers, for instance), sour, or pungent. Favor those that are mild, sweet, and bitter.

- Certain spices can inflame an already strong pitta. You can imagine the effect chili peppers and cayenne would have on you, for instance. In general, Ayurveda recommends that this dosha use spices in moderation. Some spices with cooling properties — coriander, cardamom, and fennel, to name a few — are fine.

fruits			
Friendliest	**Eat in Moderation**	**Okay if Eaten Rarely**	**Avoid**
Apples (sweet)	Limes	Kiwi	Apples (sour)
Applesauce	Papaya		Apricots (sour)
Apricots (sweet)			Bananas
Avocados			Berries (sour)
Berries (sweet)			Cherries (sour)
Cherries (sweet)			Cranberries
Coconut			Grapefruit
Dates			Grapes (green)
Figs			Lemons
Grapes (red and purple)			Mangoes (green)
Mangoes (ripe)			Olives (green)
Melons			Oranges (sour)
Olives (black)			Peaches
Oranges (sweet)			Persimmons
Pears			Pineapple (sour)
Pineapple (sweet)			Plums (sour)
Pomegranates			Rhubarb
Prunes			Strawberries
Raisins			Tamarind
Watermelon			

vegetables			
Friendliest	Eat in Moderation	Okay if Eaten Rarely	Avoid
Artichoke	Carrots (raw)	Corn	Beet greens
Asparagus		Eggplant	Beets (raw)
Beets (cooked)		Kohlrabi	Daikon radish
Broccoli		Spinach (cooked)	Garlic
Brussels sprouts			Green chilies
Cabbage			Horseradish
Carrots (cooked)			Mustard greens
Cauliflower			Onions (raw)
Celery			Peppers (hot)
Cilantro			Radishes
Cucumber			Spinach (raw)
Fennel			Tomatoes
Green beans			Turnip greens
Jerusalem artichoke			Turnips
Kale			
Leafy greens			
Lettuce			
Okra			
Parsley			
Parsnips			
Peas			
Peppers (sweet)			
Potatoes (white)			
Sweet potatoes			

legumes		
Friendliest	**Okay Once in a While**	**Avoid**
Adzuki beans	Soy flour	Soy sauce
Black beans	Soy powder	Tur dal (split
Black-eyed peas		yellow lentils)
Chickpeas (gar-		Urad dal (split
banzo beans)		black lentils)
Kidney beans		
Lentils (brown		
and red)		
Lima beans		
Mung beans		
(whole bean)		
Mung dal (split		
mung bean)		
Navy beans		
Peas (dried)		
Pinto beans		
Soybeans		
Soy cheese		
Soy milk		
Split peas		
Tofu		
White beans		

dairy products		
Friendliest	**Okay Once in a While**	**Avoid**
Butter (unsalted) Cheese (soft, not aged, unsalted) Cottage cheese Cow's milk Ghee Goat cheese (soft and unsalted) Goat's milk Ice cream	Yogurt (freshly made and diluted)	Butter (salted) Buttermilk Cheese (hard) Sour cream Yogurt (plain, frozen, or with fruit)

grains		
Friendliest	**Okay if Eaten Rarely**	**Avoid**
Amaranth	Muesli	Bread (with yeast)
Barley	Polenta	Buckwheat
Cereal (dry)	Rice (brown)	Corn
Couscous		Millet
Crackers		Oats
Durum wheat		Quinoa
flour		Rye
Granola		
Oat bran		
Oats (cooked)		
Pancakes		
Pasta		
Rice (basmati,		
white, wild)		
Rice cakes		
Sago		
Spelt		
Tapioca		
Wheat		
Wheat bran		

beverages		
Friendliest	**Drink in Moderation**	**Avoid**
Almond milk	Chai (hot spiced milk)	Apple cider
Aloe vera juice	Cinnamon tea	Berry juice (sour)
Apple juice	Orange juice	Caffeinated beverages
Apricot juice		Carbonated drinks
Berry juice (sweet)		Carrot juice
Black tea		Cherry juice (sour)
Blackberry tea		Chocolate milk
Chamomile tea		Coffee
Cherry juice (sweet)		Cranberry juice
Cool dairy drinks		Ginger tea (dry)
Grain "coffee"		Ginseng tea
Grape juice		Grapefruit juice
Mango juice		Iced drinks
Mixed vegetable juice		Iced tea
Peach nectar		Lemonade
Pear juice		Papaya juice
Pomegranate juice		Sour juices
Prune juice		Tomato juice
Rice milk		
Soy milk		
Vegetable bouillon		

nuts	
Friendliest	**Avoid**
Almonds (soaked and peeled)	Almonds (with skin) Black walnuts Brazil nuts Cashews Hazelnuts Macadamia nuts Pecans Pine nuts Pistachios Walnuts

seeds		
Friendliest	**Okay Once in a While**	**Avoid**
Flax Popcorn (no salt, buttered) Psyllium Sunflower	Pumpkin	Sesame

spices, herbs, and condiments

Friendliest	Okay in Moderation	Avoid	
Basil (fresh)	Black pepper	Ajwain	Oregano
Chutney, mango (sweet)	Caraway	Allspice	Paprika
	Cardamom	Almond extract	Pickles
Cinnamon	Cilantro	Anise	Poppy seeds
Coriander	Neem leaves	Asafetida	Rosemary
Cumin	Orange peel	Basil (dried)	Sage
Curry leaves	Parsley	Bay leaf	Salt (in excess)
Dill	Tarragon	Cayenne	Soy sauce
Fennel	Vanilla	Chili peppers (dried)	Star anise
Ginger (fresh)		Chocolate	Thyme
Mint		Chutney, mango (spicy)	Vinegar
Peppermint		Cloves	
Saffron		Fenugreek	
Spearmint		Garlic	
Turmeric		Ginger (dry)	
		Kelp	
		Ketchup	
		Lemon	
		Mace	
		Marjoram	
		Mayonnaise	
		Mustard	
		Mustard seeds	
		Nutmeg	

oils		
Friendliest (for Internal and External Use)	**External Use Only**	**Avoid**
Canola Flaxseed Ghee Olive Primrose Soy Sunflower Walnut	Avocado Coconut	Almond Apricot Corn Safflower Sesame

sweeteners		
Friendliest	**Okay if Used Rarely**	**Avoid**

Barley malt
Fructose
Fruit-juice
  concentrate
Maple syrup
Rice syrup
Turbinado
	Honey (raw and
	  not processed)
	White sugar
		Jaggery
		Molasses

kapha

General Guidelines

- Low-fat milk balances kapha. Make sure you consume it in the way it should be: boiled, then cooled to room temperature. Adding a pinch or two of turmeric before boiling reduces the kapha-generating qualities of even whole milk.
- Kapha is a heavy dosha. Balance it with such light fruits as apples and pears. Stay away from heavy, juicy, sour fruits. Most vegetables are good for you, except those that are seen as "sweet" — cucumber and tomatoes, for instance.
- Kapha is already rich in "sweetness," so it does not need sugar-based products. Your sweetener of choice should be honey.
- Beans are generally good for kapha, but nuts can aggravate the heaviness of this dosha; eat them as sparingly as possible. Most grains will benefit you, but avoid eating too much wheat or rice, which can increase mucus production and make you feel heavier.
- Rejoice! There is almost no spice that you cannot consume in abundance. "Hot" spices such as cayenne and black pepper flush out mucus, thus balancing kapha. Even mild spices will help you digest and assimilate your food better.

fruits			
Friendliest	Eat in Moderation	Okay if Eaten Rarely	Avoid
Apples	Figs (dried)	Mangoes	Avocados
Applesauce	Grapes		Bananas
Apricots	Lemons		Coconut
Berries	Limes		Dates
Cherries	Strawberries		Figs (fresh)
Cranberries			Grapefruit
Peaches			Kiwi
Pears			Melons
Persimmons			Olives (black or green)
Pomegranates			Oranges
Prunes			Papaya
Raisins			Pineapple
			Plums
			Rhubarb
			Tamarind
			Watermelon

vegetables	
Friendliest	**Avoid**
Artichoke	Cucumber
Asparagus	Squash (winter)
Beet greens	Sweet potatoes
Beets	Tomatoes (raw)
Broccoli	Zucchini
Brussels sprouts	
Cabbage	
Carrots	
Cauliflower	
Celery	
Cilantro	
Corn	
Daikon radish	
Eggplant	
Fennel	
Green beans	
Green chilies	
Horseradish	
Jerusalem artichoke	
Kale	
Kohlrabi	
Leafy greens	
Lettuce	
Mustard greens	
Okra	

legumes		
Friendliest	Eat in Moderation	Avoid
Adzuki beans	Mung beans	Kidney beans
Black beans	(whole beans)	Soybeans
Black-eyed peas	Mung dal (split	Soy cheese
Chickpeas (gar-	mung bean)	Soy flour
banzo beans)	Tofu (hot)	Soy powder
Lentils (red and		Soy sauce
brown)		Tofu (cold)
Lima beans		Urad dal (split
Navy beans		black lentils)
Peas (dried)		
Pinto beans		
Soy milk		
Split peas		
Tur dal (split		
yellow lentils)		
White beans		

dairy products			
Friendliest	**Eat in Moderation**	**Okay if Eaten Rarely**	**Avoid**
Cottage cheese (from skimmed goat's milk) Goat's milk (skimmed) Yogurt (skimmed and diluted)	Buttermilk Ghee Goat cheese (unsalted and not aged)	Butter (unsalted)	Butter (salted) Cheese (soft and hard) Cow's milk Ice cream Sour cream Yogurt (plain, frozen, or with fruit)

grains			
Friendliest	Eat in Moderation	Okay if Eaten Rarely	Avoid
Barley Buckwheat Cereal (cold, dry, or puffed) Corn Couscous Crackers Granola Millet Muesli Oat bran Oats (dry) Polenta Rye Tapioca Wheat bran	Amaranth Durum wheat flour Quinoa Rice (basmati, wild) Spelt	Pasta Rice cakes	Bread (with yeast) Oats (boiled) Pancakes Rice (brown, white) Wheat

beverages		
Friendliest	**Drink in Moderation**	**Avoid**
Aloe vera juice	Apple juice	Almond milk
Apple cider	Chai (hot spiced	Carbonated drinks
Apricot juice	milk)	Cherry juice
Berry juice	Pineapple juice	(sour)
Black tea (spiced)		Chocolate milk
Blackberry tea		Coffee
Carrot juice		Cold dairy drinks
Chamomile tea		Grapefruit juice
Cherry juice		Iced tea
(sweet)		Icy cold drinks
Chicory		Lemonade
Cinnamon tea		Marshmallow tea
Cranberry juice		Orange juice
Grain "coffee"		Papaya juice
Grape juice		Rice milk
Mango juice		Sour juices
Peach nectar		Soy milk (cold)
Pear juice		Tomato juice
Pomegranate juice		
Prune juice		
Soy milk (hot and		
well-spiced)		

nuts		
Friendliest	**Okay Once in a While**	**Avoid**
Charoli	Almonds (soaked and peeled)	Black walnuts Brazil nuts Cashews Hazelnuts Macadamia nuts Pecans Pine nuts Pistachios Walnuts

seeds		
Friendliest	**Eat in Moderation**	**Avoid**
Chia Popcorn (no salt, no butter)	Flax Pumpkin Sunflower	Sesame

spices, herbs, and condiments		Okay in Moderation	Avoid
Friendliest			
Ajwain	Mustard	Fennel	Chocolate
Allspice	(without	Ketchup	Chutney,
Almond	vinegar)	Lemon	mango
extract	Mustard	Seaweed	(sweet)
Anise	seeds	Vanilla	Kelp
Asafetida	Neem leaves		Lime
Basil	Nutmeg		Mayonnaise
Bay leaf	Orange peel		Pickles
Black pepper	Oregano		Salt (in
Caraway	Paprika		excess)
Cardamom	Parsley		Soy sauce
Cayenne	Peppermint		Vinegar
Chili pep-	Poppy seeds		
pers (dried)	Rosemary		
Chutney,	Saffron		
mango	Sage		
(spicy)	Spearmint		
Cilantro	Star anise		
Cinnamon	Tarragon		
Cloves	Thyme		
Coriander	Turmeric		
Cumin			
Curry leaves			
Dill			
Fenugreek			
Ginger			
Mace			
Marjoram			
Mint			

oils			
Friendliest, but Use (Internally) in Small Amounts	External Use Only	Okay if Rarely Used	Avoid
Almond Canola Corn Ghee Sunflower	Sesame	Flaxseed	Apricot Avocado Coconut Olive Primrose Safflower Sesame (internal use) Soy Walnut

sweeteners	
Friendliest	Avoid
Fruit-juice concentrate Honey (raw and not processed)	Barley malt Fructose Jaggery Maple syrup Molasses Rice syrup Turbinado White sugar

glossary

Abhyanga: daily self-massage

Agad Tantra: toxicology

Agni: "fire," the force that governs digestion and metabolism

Ahara Shakti: appetite and digestive capacity

Akash: sky, ether

Alochaka: "critic" — the fire that can "criticize," or in another sense, "perceive" visually

Alochaka pitta: subdosha located in the eyes and governs vision

Ama: undigested toxic matter

Amla: the sour taste

Ananda: bliss

Apana: downward moving

Apana vata: subdosha that resides in the nether regions and regulates the flow of waste, ejaculate, and menstrual fluid

Arjuna: a key Ayurvedic herb that heals the emotional aspect of the heart

Artha: money; also, the responsibility to earn money

Asafetida: a strongly aromatic spice used in Indian cooking

Asana: a yoga pose

Ashwagandha: a key Ayurvedic herb that is an effective weapon against physical fatigue

Asthi: bone

Atta: chapati flour

Avalambaka kapha: from *avalamb*, "support," thus the form of water that gives support; this subdosha supports all other subdoshas and protects the heart and lungs and strengthens the muscles

Bal Chikitsa: pediatrics

Basti: herb-based enemas that are a crucial cleansing stage in panchakarma therapy

Beej-bhoomi: seedbed; in Ayurvedic terms, dosha imbalances make the body a beej-bhoomi for disease to grow

Bhakti yoga: a form of yoga that teaches how to attain bliss through worship

Bheda: last stage of disease, when it becomes chronic

Bhrajaka: means "to diffuse" or "spread"

Bhrajaka pitta: subdosha that gives the skin radiance

Bodhaka: from *bodh*, meaning "awareness"

Bodhaka kapha: from *bodh*, "awareness," therefore Bodhaka kapha means the form of water that helps us perceive taste — the first stage of digestion; this subdosha helps us discriminate strong and subtle flavors

Brahmi: a key Ayurvedic herb that enhances mental capacities

Chapati: griddle-cooked Indian bread

Charaka: the most revered Ayurvedic physician of ancient times

Charaka Samhita: Charaka's treatise on Ayurvedic healing

Chatai: straw mat

Darshana: observation; the first stage in Ayurvedic diagnosis

Dharma: religion, religious duty

Dhatu: tissue

Dhi: acquisition of knowledge

Dhriti: retention of knowledge

Dincharya: daily routine

Dosha: an individual's body and personality type

Dravyaguna: Ayurvedic pharmacology

Garam masala: a hot spice mix, available in Asian grocery stores

Ghee: clarified butter

Graha Chikitsa: psychiatry

Gunam: inner beauty

Gunas: qualities, either physical or abstract

Hatha yoga: a form of yoga in which exercises or poses called asanas are practiced

Jaggery: an unrefined brown sugar made from palm sap

Jal: water

Jatharagni: digestive fire

Jnana yoga: a form of yoga that uses the intellect to help understand the self

Kama: pleasure

Kapha: one of the three doshas; kapha is responsible for body structure

Karma: actions

Karma yoga: a form of yoga that teaches unselfish action

Kashaya: the astringent taste

Katu: the bitter taste

Kaya Chikitsa: internal medicine

Kheer: Indian rice pudding

Khichari: a rice and lentil dish

Kledaka kapha: the form of water that moistens; this subdosha controls the enzymes and juices that are involved in the digestive process

Lassi: diluted yogurt drink that aids digestion and cools the system

Lavana: the salty taste

Madhura: the sweet taste

Majja: bone marrow

Mamsa: muscle

Mantra yoga: a form of yoga that teaches how to use sound and speech to attain bliss

Marmas: 107 vital connecting points between mind and body

Matra: the quantity of food that is ideally suited to an individual

Matrakala: one-third of a second

Meda: fatty tissue

Moksha: the attainment of bliss

Mung dal: a yellow lentil that is light and nutritious

Nasya: Medicated oil used to clean the nasal passages

Nighantu: an Ayurvedic treatise

Ojas (pronounced with a hard "j"): the subtle essence of energy

Pachaka: pertaining to digestion

Pachaka pitta: from *pachan*, "digestion," subdosha that influences digestion, assimilation, and metabolization of food

Panchakarma: seasonal rejuvenation therapy that uses five cleansing actions (emesis, purgation, enemas, nasal cleansing, and blood purification) to detoxify the body

Paneer: homemade cottage cheese (Indian-style)

Pitta: the dosha that regulates metabolism

Pragya aparadh: literally "a mistake of the intellect," eg. refers to the body's innate intelligence being compromised

Prakopa: the second phase of disease, in which toxins increase and doshas are aggravated

Prakriti: the basic dosha type or constitution with which a person is born

Pramana: state of physical development in proportion to a person's age

Prana: life force, consciousness

Prana vata: from *prana*, "life force"; chief subdosha, located in the head, heart, chest, and sense organs and governs vision, hearing, smell, taste, creative thinking, and enthusiasm

Pranayama: a breathing exercise geared toward regulating life force

Prasara: the third phase of disease, in which the disease spreads throughout the body

Prashna: questioning; a step in Ayurvedic diagnosis

Prithvi: earth

Raita: a cool dish made by stirring chopped fruit or vegetables into plain whisked yogurt

Rajas: the guna or quality that moves us to take action

Raja yoga: a form of yoga that teaches royal qualities to put an end to worldly miseries and attain bliss

Rakta: blood tissue

Ranjaka: that which colors

Ranjaka pitta: subdosha that governs the liver, spleen, and stomach and gives healthy blood its rich red color

Rasa: taste; Ayurveda recognizes six primary rasas, or tastes. Taken literally, it means "essence" as well as "fluid"

Rasayana: a healing food that balances both body and mind

Rig-Veda: the oldest Indian text

Roopam: outer or physical beauty

Sadhaka: the fire that helps us recognize the truth or reality, from the root *sadh*, meaning "to accomplish" or "to realize"

Sadhaka pitta: heart-based subdosha that metabolizes thought and feeling

Sadhu: wandering mendicants who spend their days meditating, worshipping, visiting pilgrimage centers across India, and seeking alms

Samana: balance or equalizing

Samana vata: subdosha residing in the midsection of the body, including the navel, stomach, and small intestine

Samanvaya: balance

Samhanana: assessment of a person's physical build

Samhita: compilation

Sanchaya: accumulate

Sanskrit: the language of ancient India

Sara: assessment of a person's hair, skin, eyes, and voice

Sat chit ananda: purity of soul and total bliss

Satmya: assessment of a person's habits

Sattva: the highest guna, or quality of the mind

Shalakya Tantra: eye, ear, nose, and throat treatment

Shalya Tantra: surgery

Shirodhara: a luxurious step during panchakarma in which a continuous stream of oil is poured on the forehead for about thirty minutes

Shrotas: bodily channels

Shukra: reproductive

Sleshaka kapha: from the root word *slish*, which means to be moist or sticky; this subdosha is located in the joints and is responsible for their integrity and movement

Smriti: the ability to recall what has been learned

Sparsha: touch, one of the stages in an Ayurvedic diagnosis

Sthanasamsarya: the fourth stage of disease, in which toxins get localized

Susruta Samhita: an ancient treatise, mainly on surgery, written by Susruta

Swastha: the Sanskrit word for "healthy"

Swedana: an herb-infused steam bath that opens up the channels of healing during panchakarma

Tamas: one of the three behavioral doshas, associated with inaction and making unwise choices

Tantra yoga: a form of yoga that teaches how to attain bliss using certain ancient Hindu scriptures

Tarpaka: from *tripti,* "contentment"

Tarpaka kapha: derived from *tripti,* which means "contentment," thus tarpaka kapha means the form of water that gives contentment; this subdosha nourishes the nose, mouth, eyes, and brain

Tikiya: a popular potato snack in India

Tikta: the pungent taste

Tridosha: the three doshas

Turka: fried garnish

Udana: upward moving

Udana vata: subdosha responsible for quality of voice, memory, and movement of thought

Upveda: a subtext of the Vedas, ancient Indian philosophical works

Vaidya: an Ayurvedic physician

Vajikarana Tantra: study of aphrodisiacs and fertility

Vastu: Hindu philosophy of home architecture

Vata: the dosha that governs movement and leads the other two doshas

Vaya: age and its relationship with disease

Vayastyag: lasting beauty

Vayu: air

Vedas: ancient Indian texts; there are four vedas: Rig-Veda, Sama-Veda, Yajur-Veda, and Atharva-Veda

Vikriti: a person's current balance of doshas, influenced by several factors

Vyakti: the fifth phase of disease, in which it becomes evident

Vyana (vi-ana): diffusive or pervasive. *Vi* is a prefix meaning apart or to separate

Vyana vata: subdosha whose primary seat is the heart; governs blood flow, heart rhythm, perspiration, and sense of touch

Vyayama Shakti: a person's capacity to exercise and work

Yoga: a sister science of Ayurveda, designed to unite the human mind and the divine through disciplined asanas, or poses

Yuj: to join together, yoke, unite

resource list

seven informative ayurveda web sites

www.mapi.com

Maharishi Ayurveda's comprehensive Web site contains several free newsletters on Ayurveda. The topics include nutrition tips and recipes, skin-care advice, counsel on creating joyful relationships, and recommendations on maintaining overall balance. In addition, you'll find here a vaidya's advice on common health problems, plus interviews with allopathic doctors who combine their practice of Western medicine with Ayurvedic treatments.

www.discoverayurveda.com

Another good site that covers a variety of Ayurvedic topics, from yoga poses for a smooth menopause to skin-care strategies. You can also read book reviews and subscribe to free online Ayurvedic newsletters here.

www.ayurveda.com

This is the Web site of the Ayurvedic Institute in Albuquerque, New Mexico. Along with detailed information about the institute and its Ayurvedic teaching programs, you will find here articles by Dr. Vasant Lad, who has written several books on Ayurveda.

www.niam.com

This site is for the National Institute of Ayurvedic Medicine, established by Scott Gerson, M.D. The site lists and briefly explains some basic Sanskrit terms used in Ayurveda. Those who would like to go into slightly more detail on, say, the various kinds of digestive fire, or agni, will find this a useful quick-introduction guide.

www.blissful-sleep.com

For sound advice on sound sleep and stress-free living, this is a valuable Ayurvedic Web site. The site also features buying information on some herb-based Ayurvedic sleep-promoting products.

www.ayurvedic.org

Run by Pratap Chauhan, an Ayurvedic physician based in India, this Web site has a helpful section entitled "Ayurbasics."

www.mspa.com

This Web site will give you practical tips on Ayurvedic beauty care. Check out the "Weekly Wisdom" section and the article "How to Do An Abhyanga (self-massage)."

---

seven must-read ayurveda books

Gerson, Scott, M.D. *Ayurveda: The Ancient Indian Healing Art.* Boston: Element Books, 1993.

Hospodar, Miriam Kasin. *Heaven's Banquet: Vegetarian Cooking for Lifelong Health the Ayurveda Way.* New York: Dutton, 1999.

Lad, Vasant, B.A.M.S., M.A.SC. *The Complete Book of Ayurvedic Home Remedies.* New York: Harmony Books, 1998.

Lonsdorf, Nancy, M.D., Veronica Butler, M.D., and Melanie Brown, Ph.D. *A Woman's Best Medicine: Health, Happiness, and Long Life Through Ayur-Veda.* New York: Jeremy P. Tarcher/Putnam, 1993.

Raichur, Pratima, with Marian Cohn. *Absolute Beauty.* New York: Harper Collins, 1997.

Reddy, Kumuda, M.D., and Stan Kendz. *Forever Healthy:*

Introduction to Maharishi Ayurveda Health Care. Kensington, Md.: Samhita Enterprises, 1997.

Sharma, Hari, and Christopher Clark. *Contemporary Ayurveda: Medicine and Research in Ayurveda.* New York: Churchill Livingstone, 1998.

Sharma, Hari. *Freedom from Disease.* Toronto: Veda Publishing, Inc., 1993.

how you can study ayurveda

American Institute of Vedic Studies

P.O. Box 8357
Santa Fe, NM 87504-8357
Web site: www.vedanet.com
E-mail: vedicinst@aol.com
Phone: (505) 983-9385
Fax: (505) 982-5807

American University of Complementary Medicine

11543 Olympic Boulevard
Los Angeles, CA 90064
Web site: www.aucm.org
E-mail: info@aucm.org
Phone: (310) 914-4116
Fax: (310) 479-3376

The Ayurvedic Institute

11311 Menaul NE
Albuquerque, NM 87112
Web site: www.ayurveda.com
E-mail: info@ayurveda.com
Phone: (505) 291-9698
Fax: (505) 294-7572

Banaras Hindu University

Registrar
Varanasi - 221 005, India
Web site: bhu.ac.in
Phone: +91-0542-316558
Fax: +91-0542-316558

College of Maharishi Vedic Medicine

Maharishi University of Management
1000 North Fourth Street
Fairfield, IA 52557
Web site: www.mum.edu/cmvm
E-mail: admissions@mum.edu
Phone: (800) 369-6480 or (641) 472-1110
Fax: (641) 472-1179

International Centre for Ayurvedic Studies

Post Bag No. 4
Jamnagar 361008
Gujarat, India

Web site: www.ayurveduniversity.com
Phone: +91-288-677324; 676854; 558260
Fax: +91-288-555966
E-mail: Ayurveda-uni-jam@hotmail.com

how to locate a vaidya

Many people have asked me how to locate a vaidya. Let me give you contact information for two vaidyas I can personally recommend.

Vaidya Ramakant Mishra

Maharishi Ayurveda Products
1068 Elkton Drive
Colorado Springs, CO 80907
Web site: www.mapi.com
E-mail: info@mapi.com
Phone: (800) 345-8332 or (719) 260-5500
Fax: (719) 260-7400

Dr. Vasant Lad

The Ayurvedic Institute
11311 Menaul NE
Albuquerque, NM 87112
Web site: www.ayurveda.com
E-mail: info@ayurveda.com
Phone: (505) 291-9698
Fax: (505) 294-7572

Both Maharishi Ayurveda and The Ayurvedic Institute can provide you with a resource list for finding a vaidya in your area. You can also use the Internet as a resource, or you might ask trusted friends or colleagues for a recommendation.

recommended buying guide

There are many companies that sell Ayurvedic products, yet not all of them sell all-natural products. However, I can recommend some companies that are known to be reliable and reputable. Here they are:

Amrita Aromatherapy

1900 West Stone
Fairfield, IA 52556
Web site: www.amrita.net
E-mail: info@amrita.net
Phone: (641) 472-9136
Fax: (641) 472-8672

Aroma Vera

American Brand Labs
5310 Beethoven St.
Los Angeles, CA 90066
Web site: www.aromavera.com
E-mail: cservice@aromavera.com
Phone: (800) 669-9514 or (310) 574-6920
Fax: (310) 574-5873

Auromere Ayurvedic Imports

2621 West Highway 12
Lodi, CA 95242
Web site: www.auromere.com
E-mail: info@auromere.com
Phone: (800) 735-4691

Ayurvedica

P.O. Box 871
Flagstaff, AZ 86002-0871
Web site: www.ayurvedica.net
E-mail: info@ayurvedica.net
Phone: (877) 901-8332 (VEDA)

Banyan Trading Co.

P.O. Box 13002
Albuquerque, NM 87192
Web site: www.banyantrading.com
E-mail: info@banyantrading.com
Phone: (800) 953-6424

Maharishi Ayurveda

1068 Elkton Drive
Colorado Springs, CO 80907
Web site: www.mapi.com
E-mail: info@mapi.com
Phone: (800) 345-8332 or (719) 260-5500
Fax: (719) 260-7400

Essential Oil Reference Books

Lawless, Julia. *The Illustrated Encyclopedia of Essential Oils: The Complete Guide to the Use of Oils in Aromatherapy and Herbalism.* Boston: Element Books, 1995.

Rose, Jeanne. *375 Essential Oils and Hydrosols.* Berkeley, Calif.: Frog Ltd., 1999.

Schiller, David, and Carol Schiller (contributor). *500 Formulas for Aromatherapy: Mixing Essential Oils for Every Use.* New York: Sterling Publishing Co., Inc., 1994.

Worwood, Valerie Ann. *The Complete Book of Essential Oils and Aromatherapy.* Novato, Calif.: New World Library, 1991.

Herbal Teas

Check out the Maharishi Ayurveda catalog at: www.mapi.com or call them at (800) 345-8332 or (719) 260-5500, or you may e-mail them at info@mapi.com.

Tongue Cleaner or Tongue Scraper

Available online at www.mapi.com, www.evolutionhealth.com, and at most natural health stores.

index

A

affirmations, 160

age, disease and *(vaya)*, 35

ajwain, 137–38

alochaka pitta, 72

ama, 21–26; catching early, 24–26; daily routine and, 83; mental and emotional, 23–24; physical, 21–23; stress as, 164–65; yoga to detoxify, 184. *See also* toxins

apana vata, 71

appetite and digestive capacity *(ahara shakti)*, 35; keenness of, 198–99

apple: cooked, chutney, 134; gift of, 205–6; stewed, 128

asthma, 76

avalambaka kapha, 74

Ayurveda: antiquity of, xvii, 211–12; appetite, keenness of, 198–99; attendant and healing process, 32–33; awakening the doctor within you, 7–9; balance of body, mind, spirit and health, 13–26, 197–98; comprehensive texts of, 212; connection with the universe, human beings, and, 9–11; definition of healer, 29–30; eat fresh, eat red, yellow, green, 196; founding fathers, xviii; gift ideas, 202–7; live life clean, 197; medicine or herbal formulas *(dravyaguna)*, 31–32; origins, xvii; patient and, 32; power of one, 201–2; practice of, requirements for, 3; seeking serenity, 199–200; stay fit, stay lean, 196–97; stress, role of, 5–7; two steps: doing less, being more, 3, 4–5; view life clearly, 200; way, xvi

B

Bach, Richard, 195

Bailey, Pearl, 93

balance (of body, mind, spirit), 13–26, 197–98; daily routine and, 79–92; *samanvaya* (perfect), 159; *swastha* (healthy) and, 16–17; treatment oriented toward restoring, 38–39; yoga and, 181–84

261

T

U

V

about the author

Fifteen years ago, Shubhra Krishan could not have written this book. Her life was a heady mix of danger, excitement, and desperate deadlines. She was reporting for prime-time network news to 400 million viewers across India. Shubhra never had the time to care for her own health, let alone tell you how to care for yours. In the blink of an eye, her life changed the day a vaidya placed his finger on her pulse. That's when she discovered the wonder of Ayurveda.

The experience inspired her to pen a long-running series on Ayurvedic living for network television in India called *Feeling Fine.* The immensely popular weekly series focused on simple ways to live a healthy Ayurvedic lifestyle.

Shubhra worked as the multimedia editor for a successful natural products company in the United States. She is now editorial director for a Chicago-based company that produces media software on health and entertainment. Besides writing on health and lifestyle for American magazines and Web sites, she is now working on her second book. She lives with her husband, Hemant, and son, Harshvardhan, in Colorado Springs, Colorado.